Minimally Invasive Oncologic Surgery, Part II

Editors

CLAUDIUS CONRAD

JAMES W. FLESHMAN Jr

SURGICAL ONCOLOGY CLINICS OF NORTH AMERICA

www.surgonc.theclinics.com

Consulting Editor

TIMOTHY M. PAWLIK

April 2019 • Volume 28 • Number 2

ELSEVIER

1600 John F. Kennedy Boulevard • Suite 1800 • Philadelphia, Pennsylvania, 19103-2899

http://www.theclinics.com

SURGICAL ONCOLOGY CLINICS OF NORTH AMERICA Volume 28, Number 2
April 2019 ISSN 1055-3207, ISBN-13: 978-0-323-67823-0

Editor: John Vassallo (j.vassallo@elsevier.com)
Developmental Editor: Sara Watkins

Surgical Oncology Clinics of North America (ISSN 1055-3207) is published quarterly by Elsevier Inc., 360 Park Avenue South, New York, NY 10010-1710. Months of publication are January, April, July, and October. Business and Editorial Offices: 1600 John F. Kennedy Blvd., Ste. 1800, Philadelphia, PA 19103-2899. Customer Service Office: 3251 Riverport Lane, Maryland Heights, MO 63043. Periodicals postage paid at New York, NY and additional mailing offices. Subscription prices are $306.00 per year (US individuals), $533.00 (US institutions) $100.00 (US student/resident), $352.00 (Canadian individuals), $674.00 (Canadian institutions), $205.00 (Canadian student/resident), $422.00 (foreign individuals), $674.00 (foreign institutions), and $205.00 (foreign student/resident). Foreign air speed delivery is included in all *Clinics* subscription prices. All prices are subject to change without notice. **POSTMASTER**: Send address changes to *Surgical Oncology Clinics of North America,* Elsevier Health Science Division, Subscription Customer Service, 3251 Riverport Lane, Maryland Heights, MO 63043. **Customer Service: 1-800-654-2452 (US and Canada). 314-447-8871 (outside US and Canada). Fax: 314-447-8029. E-mail: journalscustomerservice-usa@elsevier.com (for print support); journalsonline support-usa@elsevier.com (for online support).**

Reprints. For copies of 100 or more, of articles in this publication, please contact the Commercial Reprints Department, Elsevier Inc., 360 Park Avenue South, New York, New York 10010-1710. Tel. 212-633-3874; Fax: 212-633-3820; E-mail: reprints@elsevier.com.

Surgical Oncology Clinics of North America is covered in *MEDLINE/PubMed (Index Medicus)* and *EMBASE/ Excerpta Medica, Current Contents/Clinical Medicine, and ISI/BIOMED.*

Contributors

CONSULTING EDITOR

TIMOTHY M. PAWLIK, MD, MPH, MTS, PhD, FACS, FRACS (Hon.)
Professor and Chair, Department of Surgery, The Urban Meyer III and Shelley Meyer
Chair for Cancer Research, Professor of Surgery, Oncology, and Health Services
Management and Policy, Surgeon in Chief, The Ohio State University, Wexner
Medical Center, Columbus, Ohio, USA

EDITORS

CLAUDIUS CONRAD, MD, PhD, FACS
Chief of General Surgery and Surgical Oncology, Saint Elizabeth's Medical Center, Tufts
University School of Medicine, Boston, Massachusetts, USA

JAMES W. FLESHMAN Jr, MD, FACS, FASCRS
Surgeon in Chief, Baylor University Medical Center, Sparkman Endowed Chair of Surgery,
Professor of Surgery, Texas A&M Health Science Center, Dallas, Texas, USA

AUTHORS

HORACIO J. ASBUN, MD, FACS
Department of General Surgery, Mayo Clinic, Jacksonville, Florida, USA; Chief of
Hepatobiliary and Pancreas Surgery, Miami Cancer Institute, Miami, Florida, USA;
Adjunct Professor of Surgery, Mayo Clinic College of Medicine and Sciences,
Rochester, Minnesota, USA

IOANA BAIU, MD, MPH
Resident, Department of Surgery, Stanford University School of Medicine, Stanford,
California, USA

JOSEPH R. BROUCEK, MD
Assistant Professor, Department of Surgery, Vanderbilt University Medical Center,
Nashville, Tennessee, USA; Department of General Surgery, Mayo Clinic, Jacksonville,
Florida, USA

SEAN P. CLEARY, MD, MSc, MPH, FRCSC
Department of Surgery, Division of Hepatobiliary Surgery, Mayo Clinic, Rochester,
Minnesota, USA

CHRISTINA L. COSTANTINO, MD
Department of Surgery, Massachusetts General Hospital, Boston, Massachusetts,
USA

LAURA M. ENOMOTO, MSc, MD
Fellow in Surgical Oncology, Wake Forest Baptist Medical Center, Winston-Salem,
North Carolina, USA

JAIRAM R. ESWARA, MD
St. Elizabeth's Hospital, Tufts University School of Medicine, Boston, Massachusetts, USA

DAVID FUKS, MD, PhD
Department of Digestive, Oncologic and Metabolic Surgery, InstitutMutualisteMontsouris, Université Paris Descartes, Paris, France

BRICE GAYET, MD, PhD
Department of Digestive, Oncologic and Metabolic Surgery, InstitutMutualisteMontsouris, Université Paris Descartes, Paris, France

DAVID A. GELLER, MD
Director, Department of Surgery, Division of Hepatobiliary and Pancreatic Surgery, UPMC Liver Cancer Center, University of Pittsburgh Medical Center, Pittsburgh, Pennsylvania, USA

STEVEN N. HOCHWALD, MD, MBA
Professor, Department of Surgical Oncology, Roswell Park Comprehensive Cancer Center, Buffalo, New York, USA

COLLEEN M. KIERNAN, MD, MPH
Fellow, Department of Surgical Oncology, The University of Texas MD Anderson Cancer Center, Houston, Texas, USA

DICKEN S. KO, MD
St. Elizabeth's Hospital, Tufts University School of Medicine, Boston, Massachusetts, USA

MOSHIM KUKAR, MD
Assistant Professor, Department of Surgical Oncology, Roswell Park Comprehensive Cancer Center, Buffalo, New York, USA

MICHAEL KUNCEWITCH, MD
Fellow in Surgical Oncology, Wake Forest Baptist Medical Center, Winston-Salem, North Carolina, USA

JEFFREY E. LEE, MD
Professor, Chair, Department of Surgical Oncology, The University of Texas MD Anderson Cancer Center, Houston, Texas, USA

EDWARD A. LEVINE, MD
Professor of Surgery, Wake Forest Baptist Medical Center, Winston-Salem, North Carolina, USA

GARY N. MANN, MD
Associate Professor, Department of Surgical Oncology, Roswell Park Comprehensive Cancer Center, Buffalo, New York, USA

JOHN T. MULLEN, MD
Department of Surgery, Massachusetts General Hospital, Associate Professor of Surgery, Harvard Medical School, Boston, Massachusetts, USA

JUNE S. PENG, MD
Fellow, Department of Surgical Oncology, Roswell Park Comprehensive Cancer Center, Buffalo, New York, USA

KATHLEEN C. PERRY, BS
Assistant Project Manager, Wake Forest Baptist Medical Center, Winston-Salem, North Carolina, USA

WALTER R. PETERS, MD, MBA
Chief, Division of Colon and Rectal Surgery, Baylor University Medical Center, Dallas, Texas, USA

DOMINIC SANFORD, MD
Department of General Surgery, Mayo Clinic, Jacksonville, Florida, USA; Assistant Professor, Department of Surgery, Barnes-Jewish Hospital, St Louis, Missouri, USA

MARCEL SANHUEZA, MD
Assistant Professor, Department of Digestive Surgery, Faculty of Medicine, Catholic University of Chile, Santiago, Chile

ANTHONY SENAGORE, MD, MBA
Professor, Department of Surgery, Western Michigan University, Homer Stryker School of Medicine, Kalamazoo, Michigan, USA

PERRY SHEN, MD, FACS
Professor of Surgery, Wake Forest Baptist Medical Center, Winston-Salem, North Carolina, USA

JOHN A. STAUFFER, MD, FACS
Department of General Surgery, Mayo Clinic, Associate Professor, Department of Surgery, The Mayo Clinic Hospital, Jacksonville, Florida, USA

FORAT SWAID, MD
Department of Surgery, Division of Hepatobiliary and Pancreatic Surgery, UPMC Liver Cancer Center, University of Pittsburgh Medical Center, Pittsburgh, Pennsylvania, USA

EDUARDO A. VEGA, MD
Postdoctoral Fellow, Department of Surgical Oncology, The University of Texas MD Anderson Cancer Center, Houston, Texas, USA; Department of Surgery, Hepato-bilio-pancreatic Surgery Unit, Hospital Sotero Del Rio, Santiago, Chile

EDUARDO VIÑUELA, MD
Assistant Professor, Department of Digestive Surgery, Faculty of Medicine, Catholic University of Chile, Santiago, Chile; Assistant Professor of Surgery, Department of Digestive Surgery, Faculty of Medicine, Catholic University of Chile, Sotero del Rio Hospital, Puente Alto, Chile

BRENDAN C. VISSER, MD
Associate Professor, Department of Surgery, Stanford University School of Medicine, Stanford, California, USA

KONSTANTINOS I. VOTANOPOULOS, MD, PhD, FACS
Associate Professor of Surgery, Wake Forest Baptist Medical Center, Winston-Salem, North Carolina, USA

KATERINA O. WELLS, MD, MPH
Adjunct Assistant Professor, Texas A&M Health Sciences, Director of Colorectal Research, Department of Surgery, Division of Colon and Rectal Surgery, Baylor University Medical Center, Dallas, Texas, USA

LAVANYA YOHANATHAN, MD
Department of Surgery, Division of Hepatobiliary Surgery, Mayo Clinic, Rochester, Minnesota, USA

Contents

Cytoreductive surgery (CRS) and hyperthermic intraperitoneal chemotherapy (HIPEC) is an evolving strategy in the locoregional management of peritoneal surface malignancies, and the role of laparoscopy is expanding. Staging laparoscopy is routinely used to obtain tissue for diagnosis and assess extent of tumor burden. Laparoscopic CRS and HIPEC with curative intent is safe and effective in patients with a low disease burden. In patients with refractory malignant ascites, complete resolution of ascites and improvement in quality of life have been demonstrated with palliative laparoscopic HIPEC. Laparoscopic CRS and HIPEC has an expanding role in the treatment of peritoneal surface disease.

Laparoscopic and thoracoscopic or robotic-assisted minimally invasive esophagectomy offers benefits in decreased postoperative complications and faster recovery. The choice of operation depends on patient and surgeon factors. McKeown or 3-field esophagectomy requires dissection in the abdomen, chest, and neck, with a cervical anastomosis. Ivor Lewis esophagectomy is performed with abdominal and right chest dissection and intrathoracic anastomosis. Transhiatal or transmediastinal esophagectomy is performed with abdominal and cervical dissections and a cervical anastomosis and is preferential in patients with significant pulmonary risk factors. Preparation and operative conduct for laparoscopic and robotic approaches for these operations, and the expected postoperative recovery are detailed.

Minimally invasive surgical approaches to the treatment of gastric cancer have become increasingly common as more data have demonstrated the safety, feasibility, and oncologic equivalency of such approaches compared with conventional open gastrectomy. East Asia has produced the majority of these data, encouraging Western high-volume centers to expand their application of minimally invasive techniques to patients despite more advanced tumor stages at presentation and a lower volume of cases. More randomized, controlled trials and longer term outcome data are necessary to definitively establish the superiority of minimally invasive gastrectomy to open gastrectomy for the treatment of gastric cancer.

Laparoscopic liver resection (LLR) for hepatocellular carcinoma (HCC) has been rapidly expanding. With increasing experience, the safety and feasibility of LLR for HCC have been demonstrated. LLR of HCC is becoming the standard of care for minor liver resections, and even major LLR are being performed safely in experienced centers. In most reports, patients undergoing LLR had less blood loss, fewer transfusions, less postoperative morbidity, and shorter length of stay compared with open liver resections (OLR). The 5-year overall and disease-free survival rates for patients undergoing LLR for HCC are comparable to OLR.

Laparoscopic liver surgery for secondary liver cancer is increasing. The most common indications are colorectal cancer liver metastases followed by adenocarcinoma metastases from other solid organs, such as breast, pancreatic neuroendocrine, and other gastrointestinal tract cancers. This article provides a comprehensive review of crucial concepts when managing secondary liver cancer minimally invasively, a summary of the up-to-date literature, and a discussion of the development of the application of this technique over time.

 Video content accompanies this article at http://www.surgonc. theclinics.com.

There is consensus that oncologic extended resection should be performed for resectable incidental and nonincidental gallbladder cancer. The safety and feasibility of a minimally invasive approach to oncologic extended resection of gallbladder cancer has been demonstrated and is performed in centers of expertise worldwide. In this article, a systematic approach to the indications and techniques for a minimally invasive approach to extended resection for gallbladder cancer is detailed.

In pancreatic cancer, resection combined with neoadjuvant and/or adjuvant therapy remains the only chance for cure and/or prolonged survival. A minimally invasive approach to pancreatic cancer has gained increased acceptance and popularity. The aim of minimally invasive surgery of the pancreas includes limiting trauma, decreasing length of hospitalization, lessening cost, decreasing blood loss, and allowing for a more meticulous oncologic dissection. New advances and routine use in practice have helped progress the field making the minimally invasive approach more feasible. In this article, the minimally invasive surgical approaches to proximal, central, and distal pancreatic cancer are described and literature reviewed.

Ioana Baiu and Brendan C. Visser

Small bowel malignancies are extremely rare. Surgical resection is often the mainstay of treatment with the extent of the operation depending on the type of tumor. Whereas neuroendocrine tumors and adenocarcinoma require lymph node resection, gastrointestinal stromal tumors do not typically metastasize to regional nodes and therefore need resection only. Minimally invasive approaches are applicable to small tumors that require a limited resection and reconstruction and have been shown to have equal survival benefits with decreased risk of postoperative complications.

Katerina O. Wells and Anthony Senagore

Colon cancer is the second leading cause of cancer death in the United States. Advances in surgical resection techniques, including minimally invasive colectomy, are becoming a standard of care. The oncologic principles of colectomy have included adequate lymphadenectomy, proximal ligation of primary vessels, and resection with adequate longitudinal margins. More recently, complete mesocolic excision has been advocated. Open and minimally invasive approaches must accomplish the same outcomes. This article focuses on the surgical principles of colon cancer, perioperative considerations, and technical aspects of minimally invasive colectomy. We review the current literature regarding oncologic and short-term outcomes of minimally invasive surgery.

Katerina O. Wells and Walter R. Peters

Total mesorectal excision (TME) can be safely performed through a minimally invasive approach by experienced surgeons and may offer patients benefit in certain short-term outcomes. Long-term oncologic outcomes and meta-analysis of the most recent randomized controlled trials may offer additional clarity regarding the role of laparoscopic TME and those patients for whom the approach is most appropriate. Until then, laparoscopic TME should be used judiciously. As the landscape of rectal cancer surgery evolves, the necessary constant needs to be multidisciplinary oversight of rectal cancer surgery performed by surgeons and surgical centers experienced in this critically important procedure.

Colleen M. Kiernan and Jeffrey E. Lee

Since the first description of laparoscopic adrenalectomy (LA) for pheochromocytoma and Cushing syndrome in 1992, the utilization of and indications for a minimally invasive approach to the adrenal gland have vastly expanded. Although minimally invasive adrenalectomy has been established as the preferred approach for patients with benign tumors of the adrenal gland, minimally invasive adrenalectomy for cancer remains controversial. In this article, the authors review the indications for minimally invasive adrenalectomy for adrenal nodules suspicious for, or established to represent, a primary malignancy or a site of metastatic cancer.

Urologists were early adopters of minimally invasive, specifically robotic, techniques for cancer surgery. The current trends show increasing adoption of robotic surgery for renal, bladder, and prostate cancer. Several randomized controlled trials show that robotic urologic surgery has outcomes that are at least as good as, if not superior to, open surgery.

Despite significant improvements over the last several decades in multimodality treatment for cancer, the physical removal of solid tumors via surgery continues to be the primary method of curative intent treatment. Currently, neoadjuvant treatments using modern chemotherapy and novel radiation protocols are used to reduce tumor size or diminish the risk of systemic relapse before removal of the bulk tumor. Aiming for cure, these improvements in the management of solid cancers remain dependent on the ability to remove tumors. It should always be kept in mind that progress in health care is not about "novelty" or "innovation" itself but about improvement in care or lower costs.

SURGICAL ONCOLOGY
CLINICS OF NORTH AMERICA

SERIES OF RELATED INTEREST

Surgical Clinics of North America
http://www.surgical.theclinics.com
Thoracic Surgery Clinics
http://www.thoracic.theclinics.com
Advances in Surgery
http://www.advancessurgery.com

THE CLINICS ARE AVAILABLE ONLINE!
Access your subscription at:
www.theclinics.com

SURGICAL ONCOLOGY
CLINICS OF NORTH AMERICA

Foreword

Minimally Invasive Oncologic Surgery, Part II

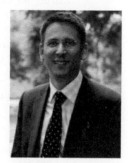

Timothy M. Pawlik, MD, MPH, MTS, PhD, FACS, FRACS (Hon.)
Consulting Editor

This issue of the *Surgical Oncology Clinics of North America* represents the second part in our series examining advances and innovations concerning surgical techniques around oncologic surgery. Given the importance, as well as expanding indications for minimally invasive oncologic surgery, we decided to dedicate two issues of *Surgical Oncology Clinics of North America* to this important topic. As with the first issue, Claudius Conrad and James Fleshman from Saint Elizabeth's Medical Center and Baylor Scott and White, respectively, acted as our esteemed guest editors. Both Dr Conrad and Dr Fleshman are well recognized and have published extensively on the topic of minimally invasive surgery (MIS), particularly as it relates to the treatment of malignant diseases. In their role as guest editors, Dr Conrad and Dr Fleshman did a wonderful job identifying world experts to write definitive, state-of-the-art articles on the application of MIS techniques to treat a wide range of cancers.

This issue of *Surgical Oncology Clinics of North America* covers a broad range of cancers including, among others, esophageal, pancreatic, liver, as well as colorectal cancer. While only a decade ago, the possibility of performing complicated procedures, such as MIS or robotic esophagectomy, pancreaticoduodenectomy, or low rectal resection, was deemed either not possible or feasible only at very select institutions, these procedures are now performed at multiple institutions throughout the United States. Despite the expanding adoption of the minimally invasive approach to these cancers, procedural details and detailed data on perioperative and long-term outcomes are still being defined. The current issue provides a comprehensive overview of these topics pertaining to minimally invasive oncological surgery related to multiple different malignancies. Thank you to Dr Conrad, Dr Fleshman, and their fantastic group

Surg Oncol Clin N Am 28 (2019) xiii–xiv
https://doi.org/10.1016/j.soc.2019.01.002
1055-3207/19/© 2019 Published by Elsevier Inc.

surgonc.theclinics.com

of contributors for an outstanding issue of the *Surgical Oncology Clinics of North America* on such an important topic.

Timothy M. Pawlik, MD, MPH, MTS, PhD, FACS, FRACS (Hon.)
Professor and Chair
Department of Surgery
The Urban Meyer III and Shelley Meyer
Chair for Cancer Research
The Ohio State University
Wexner Medical Center
395 West 12th Avenue, Suite 670
Columbus, OH 43210, USA

E-mail address:
tim.pawlik@osumc.edu

Preface

Minimally Invasive Oncologic Surgery, Part II

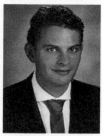
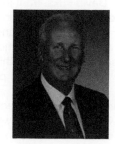

Claudius Conrad, MD, PhD, FACS   James W. Fleshman Jr, MD, FACS, FASCRS

Editors

Vision is the art of seeing the invisible.

—*Jonathan Swift*

After an exciting first issue devoted to Minimally Invasive Management of Cancer, this second issue of *Surgical Oncology Clinics of North America* expands upon innovating the treatment of cancers that were previously considered unamendable to a minimally invasive approach, including peritoneal surface, esophagogastric, and hepatopancreatobiliary (HPB) malignancies.

Working in the field of minimally invasive HPB surgery has allowed me to draw on friends who are world-renowned experts in the field. David Geller, Horacio Asbun, and Sean Cleary provide clear and comprehensive summaries of what one needs to know about HPB cancers. Eduardo A. Vega and Eduardo Viñuela, true experts in the minimally invasive management of gallbladder cancer, provide a detailed article on this rare disease, which is accompanied by multimedia content that allows the readers to experience high-quality laparoscopic management of gallbladder cancer from a unique perspective.

Furthermore, this comprehensive issue would not be complete without an expert review on the minimally invasive management of small bowel, colon, and rectal cancer. The safety and feasibility of a minimally invasive approach to colorectal cancer have been studied in landmark randomized controlled trials (MRC CLASSIC and COLOR II), which have set a high standard for the scientific assessment of the technique for other gastrointestinal cancers. In parallel, well-balanced articles on the minimally invasive management of adrenal lesions and urologic cancers show the horizontal scope of this assessment across disciplines. While Urologists have been drivers of laparoscopic

Surg Oncol Clin N Am 28 (2019) xv–xvii
https://doi.org/10.1016/j.soc.2019.01.001
1055-3207/19/© 2019 Published by Elsevier Inc.

surgonc.theclinics.com

and robotic approaches for the management of abdominal cancers, concerns regarding cost and the overall necessity of performing these operations have emerged. In this arena, Urologists are once again at the forefront of assessing value-based health care in the context of minimally invasive management of cancers. This conversation, of course, is important for all of us to have in the collective effort to move this field forward.

Finally, the editorial team is honored by the expertise of Professor Brice Gayet, together with Professor David Fuks, from Institut Mutualiste Montsouris, who provide a comprehensive and forward-looking Afterword. Brice Gayet is considered one of the pioneers of minimally invasive hepatopancreatobiliary surgery and a significantly experienced digestive disease surgeon who has tremendously advanced the field of the gastrointestinal diseases covered in this second issue. I can assure the reader of this because I have had the privilege of personally learning from him as a surgeon and a scholar.

I personally hope very much that the second issue of Minimally Invasive Management of Cancer, along with the first issue, will serve as a snapshot of today and a preamble to tomorrow as an informative, inspiring, and comprehensive learning tool for surgeons. I also would like to take the opportunity to thank again Tim Pawlik for his determined enthusiasm and support, Jim Fleshman for his help in getting this second part across the finish line, Sara Watkins for her shades of gentle reminders, and John Vassallo for his willingness to deviate from some stylistic traditions of *Surgical Oncology Clinics of North America* to allow this issue to reflect the innovative subjects within its pages.

Sincerely,

Claudius Conrad, MD, PhD, FACS

Minimally invasive techniques for the management of intra-abdominal cancer have become an accepted option for almost all solid tumors. Some of these approaches have been vetted with prospective trials, some even randomized, but it is unusual to find a discussion that encompasses all in one publication. It was this reason that led to these two-part *Surgical Oncology Clinics of North America* issues that contain discussions of almost every solid intra-abdominal tumor. The experts who have participated are experienced with both open and minimally invasive approaches, and they understand the issues that arise when making recommendations for treatment of curable cancer with new techniques. Dr Conrad and I are indebted to them for their truly authoritative contributions. The discussion around limitations of a technique is almost more important than the assumed possibilities and the recovery outcomes beyond cancer cure. As the advanced techniques are applied in institutions beyond academic institutions where clinical trials are underway, the most important consideration becomes whether generalization of the technique is possible or even appropriate.

As one reads this compilation of articles, it is hoped that a balanced message will be apparent, and that the thoughtful application of surgical judgment will be enhanced by the contents herein. Each year brings more applications for minimally invasive surgery regardless of the specific technique. The current level of application of minimally invasive techniques to cancer shows that we have the opportunity to expand their use for even the most basic and appropriate indications. Educators involved in the continued education of surgical trainees and practicing surgeons should be able to use the articles within this issue to engage trainees in a thoughtful approach to expand their use of minimally invasive surgery for resection of cancer. I would like to recognize

Dr Claudius Conrad for his incredible effort to make this publication successful and thank Dr Tim Pawlik for recognizing the need for the project.
  Respectfully,
  James W. Fleshman Jr, MD, FACS, FASCRS

Claudius Conrad, MD, PhD, FACS
Chief, General Surgery and Surgical Oncology
Director, Hepato-Pancreato-Biliary Surgery
Saint Elizabeth's Medical Center
Tufts University School of Medicine
11 Nevins Street, Suite 201
Brighton, MA 02135, USA

James W. Fleshman Jr, MD, FACS, FASCRS
Department of Surgery
Baylor University Medical Center
Texas A&M Health Science Center
3500 Gaston Avenue
1st Floor Roberts Hospital
Dallas, TX 75246, USA

E-mail addresses:
claudius.conrad@steward.org (C. Conrad)
james.fleshman@bswhealth.org (J.W. Fleshman)

Minimally Invasive Surgical Approaches for Peritoneal Surface Malignancy

Laura M. Enomoto, MSc, MD, Edward A. Levine, MD,
Kathleen C. Perry, BS, Konstantinos I. Votanopoulos, MD, PhD,
Michael Kuncewitch, MD, Perry Shen, MD*

KEYWORDS

- Peritoneal surface malignancy • Peritoneal carcinomatosis
- Hyperthermic intraperitoneal chemotherapy • Staging laparoscopy
- Laparoscopic cytoreductive surgery • Refractory malignant ascites

KEY POINTS

- Cytoreductive surgery and hyperthermic intraperitoneal chemotherapy improves survival and palliates symptoms in patients with advanced cancers with peritoneal surface disease.
- Owing to the high morbidity of open cytoreductive surgery and hyperthermic intraperitoneal chemotherapy, laparoscopic cytoreductive surgery and hyperthermic intraperitoneal chemotherapy have been proposed for selected patients with peritoneal surface malignancy.
- Staging laparoscopy is indicated to obtain biopsies and calculate a peritoneal cancer index if a diagnosis has not been previously secured.
- Laparoscopic cytoreductive surgery and hyperthermic intraperitoneal chemotherapy with curative intent may be performed safely in patients with low volume disease (peritoneal cancer index of ≤ 10).
- Palliative laparoscopic hyperthermic intraperitoneal chemotherapy are indicated in patients with refractory malignant ascites.

INTRODUCTION

Peritoneal surface malignancy defines an advanced stage in many cancers. In this context, cytoreductive surgery (CRS) and hyperthermic intraperitoneal chemotherapy

---

Disclosure Statement: None of the authors have any relationship with a commercial company that has a direct financial interest in subject matter or materials discussed in the article or with a company making a competing product.
Department of Surgery, Wake Forest Baptist Medical Center, Medical Center Boulevard, Winston Salem, NC 27157, USA
* Corresponding author.
E-mail address: pshen@wakehealth.edu

(HIPEC) have been shown to improve survival as well as palliate symptoms in patients with peritoneal surface malignancies of gastrointestinal, peritoneal, or gynecologic origin.[1–7] This therapy, however, requires an extensive abdominal incision to facilitate the evaluation and resection of all disease in the abdomen and pelvis and is associated with significant morbidity and mortality as well as a prolonged length of stay.[8] As indications for laparoscopic surgery continue to expand to include more complex and technically challenging procedures, laparoscopic CRS and HIPEC have been proposed as an option in highly selected patients to decrease the morbidity of an extensive incision and decrease prolonged hospitalizations. This article discusses the diagnosis and assessment of tumor burden of patients with peritoneal surface malignancies as well as the indications and methods of treatment using a laparoscopic approach.

DIAGNOSIS AND STAGING

Successful treatment of peritoneal surface malignancy requires a comprehensive management plan often involving perioperative systemic chemotherapy in addition to CRS and HIPEC. Diagnosis and clinical assessment of the disease burden is imperative in determining patients most likely to have a long-term benefit from treatment. Sugarbaker and Chang[9] reported 4 clinical criteria essential in evaluating patients for potential treatment and determining prognosis. First, the histopathology of the malignancy must be determined to assess the invasive nature of the disease. Second, a computed tomography (CT) scan of the chest, abdomen, and pelvis is vital for determining extent of disease and evaluating for distant metastasis. Third, calculation of the peritoneal cancer index (PCI) must be made and will influence treatment strategy. Last, determination of the completeness of cytoreduction (CC) score or residual tumor (R status) after resection becomes important for prognosis (**Box 1**).

Box 1
Essential clinical criteria

- Histopathology
- Computed tomography scan of the chest, abdomen, and pelvis
- Calculation of the peritoneal cancer index
- Determination of completeness of cytoreduction

Histopathology

Patients with peritoneal surface malignancy are often discovered on exploration for another suspected diagnosis, such as acute appendicitis or nondisseminated colon cancer. In many cases, tissues biopsies have already been obtained and can be evaluated for tumor type, grade, and invasiveness. In patients in whom peritoneal surface disease is suspected but biopsy has not yet been performed, securing a histopathologic diagnosis either through percutaneous or laparoscopic biopsy is imperative for determining treatment options. Treatment for 2 conditions—mucinous appendiceal malignancies and peritoneal mesothelioma—are particularly dependent on histopathology. Low-grade mucinous appendiceal mucinous neoplasms (disseminated peritoneal adenomucinosis, pseudomyxoma peritonei) and peritoneal mesothelioma with a nuclear diameter of less than 31 millimicrons (well-differentiated) may have extensive peritoneal spread and yet still be completely resectable.[9] Additionally, they are unlikely to metastasize to lymph nodes or other distant sites. Thus, curative intent treatment protocols may still be appropriate, even with widespread peritoneal disease.

Preoperative Imaging

A preoperative CT scan of the chest, abdomen, and pelvis is a necessity for treatment planning, with MRI of the abdomen and pelvis being an alternative. The first role is in evaluating for distant disease, because the presence of extraabdominal metastasis is a clear contraindication for CRS and HIPEC. A CT scan is also used for identifying unresectable disease. Extensive infiltration of small bowel loops and its mesentery, involvement of the ligament of Treitz, porta hepatis, lesser sac, or suprahepatic veins that would not allow for adequate cytoreduction, would be a contraindication for HIPEC.[10] Biliary and urinary obstruction are relative contraindications as well.

In patients with potentially resectable disease, preoperative CT scanning or MRI is useful for localizing and quantifying the degree of peritoneal surface disease. Nodular or plaque lesions show various levels of enhancement with intravenous contrast, and identification often depends on anatomic location.[11] Small lesions (<5 mm) are more easily distinguished on the surfaces of the liver or spleen. Lesions on curved surfaces such as the diaphragm and paracolic gutters often require image visualization on different planes.[11] Peritoneal disease from nonmucinous gastrointestinal malignancies is unfortunately not well-visualized on CT scanning because its shape often conforms to the normal contours of the abdominopelvic structures rather than distorting local structures, especially on the surface of the small bowel or colon and its mesentery.[12]

Widespread mesenteric involvement often seems to be sclerotic, with a thickened or retracted appearance. Involvement of the greater omentum, or omental caking, can appear as a thick layer of heterogenous density between the bowel and abdominal wall.[11] Bowel loops can be warped or tethered to each other, indicating bowel or mesentery involvement, even when disease is not readily apparent. Free or entrapped ascites is found in more than 70% of cases.[11] Pseudomyxoma peritonei appears as hypodense, heterogenous tissue usually around the lateral peritoneum, which may seem to be thickened owing to the irritation of the mucin itself (**Figs. 1** and **2**).

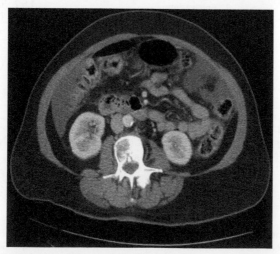

Fig. 1. Pseudomyxoma peritonei in the lateral peritoneum.

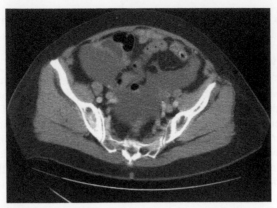

Fig. 2. Pseudomyxoma in the pelvis.

Peritoneal Cancer Index

Although there are several classifications to quantify peritoneal disease burden, the most widely used and accepted is the PCI. In this system, the abdomen is divided into 9 regions by 2 transverse planes and 2 sagittal planes (**Fig. 3**). The regions are numbered in a clockwise fashion with 0 at the umbilicus and 1 encompassing the space beneath the right diaphragm. The small bowel is divided into 4 regions (upper and lower jejunum, upper and lower ileum) and numbered 9 to 12. Each region is then assigned a lesion size (LS) score based on the amount of disease present. No macroscopic tumor present is assigned an LS of 0. If the maximum diameter of the lesions is less than 5 mm, the region is given an LS of 1. Tumor with a maximum diameter greater than 5 mm but less than 5 cm is assigned LS of 2, and any tumor greater than 5 cm or confluence is given an LS of 3. The total score for all 13 regions is the PCI, with a minimum of 0 and maximum of 39. The importance of quantifying the PCI at the beginning of the case cannot be overestimated.

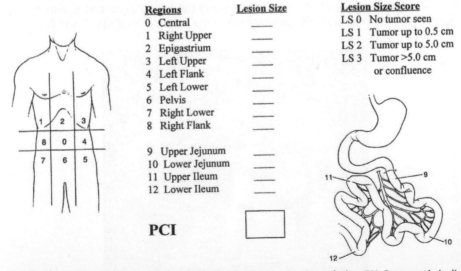

Regions	Lesion Size
0　Central	____
1　Right Upper	____
2　Epigastrium	____
3　Left Upper	____
4　Left Flank	____
5　Left Lower	____
6　Pelvis	____
7　Right Lower	____
8　Right Flank	____
9　Upper Jejunum	____
10　Lower Jejunum	____
11　Upper Ileum	____
12　Lower Ileum	____

Lesion Size Score
LS 0　No tumor seen
LS 1　Tumor up to 0.5 cm
LS 2　Tumor up to 5.0 cm
LS 3　Tumor >5.0 cm
　　　　or confluence

PCI

Fig. 3. The peritoneal cancer index (PCI). (*From* Harmon RL, Sugarbaker PH. Prognostic indicators in peritoneal carcinomatosis from gastrointestinal cancer. Int Semin Surg Oncol 2005;2(1):3; with permission.)

Completeness of Cytoreduction

A determination of residual tumor after cytoreduction is important for prognosis and treatment. There are 2 commonly used scoring systems for CC; the CC score and the residual disease score (R score) from the American Joint Committee on Cancer staging manual.[13] Numerous groups have demonstrated prognostic value of calculating a CC score in peritoneal surface disease from appendiceal, colorectal, and gastric cancers.[1,2,14–17] When no peritoneal disease is seen after cytoreduction, a CC score of 0 is assigned. A CC score of 1 indicates peritoneal nodules less than 2.5 mm in diameter remaining after cytoreduction. A CC score of 2 is assigned if nodules are between 2.5 mm and 2.5 cm, and a CC score of 3 indicates nodules greater than 2.5 cm or confluence of unresectable tumor. CC scores of 0 and 1 are considered a complete cytoreduction because a CC-1 tumor size is thought to be penetrable by intraperitoneal chemotherapy.[18]

An alternative method of quantifying residual disease is by resection margin. After cytoreduction, an R0 resection is considered complete macroscopic resection with negative margins on final pathology.[13] Complete macroscopic resection with positive microscopic margins is classified as R1. An R2 resection is considered an incomplete macroscopic resection, and is subdivided on the basis of maximal size of residual disease (R2a ≤5 mm, R2b 5 mm–20 cm, R2c >2 cm). R0 and R1 resections are considered complete cytoreductions.

INDICATIONS FOR LAPAROSCOPIC TREATMENT

Once peritoneal surface malignancy is suspected through biopsy, previous surgery or preoperative imaging, a treatment modality must be selected and tailored to the clinical picture (**Box 2**). Laparoscopy may be considered for 3 indications: staging, treatment of peritoneal surface disease, and palliative treatment of malignant ascites.

Box 2
Indications for laparoscopy in peritoneal surface malignancy

- Staging and biopsy
- Curative intent
- Palliation of malignant ascites

Staging Laparoscopy

Indications

Staging laparoscopy is often used in patients in whom a histopathologic diagnosis has not yet been made but peritoneal surface disease is suspected (**Box 3**). These patients often have undergone a CT scan of the abdomen and pelvis for nonspecific abdominal complaints or another suspected diagnosis and peritoneal disease is subsequently seen on imaging. Staging laparoscopy allows for tissue sampling of any lesions, cytologic analysis of ascites, and potentially determination of a primary source.

In patients with a known histopathologic diagnosis, staging laparoscopy is often routinely used to determine a true PCI and assess disease burden. Although a preoperative CT scan is imperative for estimation of disease and exclusion of distant metastatic or unresectable disease, many studies have demonstrated its failure to detect all peritoneal malignancy. In a study conducted by Jacquet and colleagues,[12] the sensitivity of CT a scan in determining disease was 70% to 88%, depending on the region of the abdomen. Moreover, the false-negative rate ranged from 20% to 28%. An additional study by Denzer and colleagues[19] showed peritoneal surface disease in 100% of patients with a wide range of histologically proven malignancy in whom an earlier CT showed only 47.8% with peritoneal disease.

Box 3
Indications for staging laparoscopy

- Staging and biopsy of peritoneal surface malignancy of unknown origin
- Staging of already diagnosed peritoneal surface disease
- Restaging after neoadjuvant chemotherapy

Laparoscopy can also be indicated for restaging of disease after neoadjuvant treatment. Biopsies from residual lesions or previous tumor sites can demonstrate response to treatment, and inspection of the abdomen can help to determine resectability and the PCI.

Staging laparoscopy is a relatively safe procedure, certainly with a lower morbidity than traditional laparotomy. Garofalo and Valle[20] reported a 2.1% complication rate, and no neoplastic seeding of port sites has been reported.[21] However, Garofalo and Valle[20] did find that laparoscopy understaged the degree of peritoneal disease in 2.0% of cases. At our institution, although unusual, we have encountered cases of port site recurrences.

Technique

Multiple methods of staging laparoscopy have been described. Hirano and colleagues[22] described a 3-port configuration, with a 12-mm port placed 2 cm superior to the umbilicus and 2 other 12-mm ports in the right upper and left lower quadrants. A suction cannula was used to evacuate thick, gelatinous ascites and send for culture and cytology. Biopsy specimens were routinely obtained from the peritoneum, omentum, and ovaries, and the PCI calculated. Garofalo and Valle[20] described initial Hasson trocar placement in the left or right iliac fossa on the midxillary line. They preferred not to position the trocar in the midline owing to a high incidence of adhesions from previous surgery or the tumor mass itself. Access to the iliac fossa also allowed for better visualization in the presence of an omental cake. A second 5-mm port was often placed in the contralateral iliac fossa, which was convenient for raising an omental cake. Extensive adhesiolysis was not performed, conducting only enough to calculate a PCI. Mucinous ascites was evacuated by suction, sometimes requiring upsizing of the 5-mm port to allow for a larger suction cannula. Multiple biopsies were obtained from any parietal, omental, or pelvic cavity lesions.[11]

Personal experience and results

At our institution, we prefer entry through a 5-mm Optiview trocar in the left upper quadrant as long as preoperative CT imaging does not show dense adhesions or tumor involvement at the abdominal wall in this area. Additional 5-mm ports are placed under direct vision based on the location of the initially visualized tumor burden. If thick gelatinous ascites is present, a 5-mm port may be upsized to a 12-mm trocar to allow for a larger suction cannula. Mucinous ascites is sent for cytology in addition to biopsies of any peritoneal, omental, or other suspicious lesions. A thorough inspection of the abdomen and pelvis, as well as a calculation of the PCI is always undertaken. Although some institutions proceed immediately to CRS and HIPEC, we typically perform laparoscopy in a staged fashion. This way, if the patient is not found to be a candidate for CRS and HIPEC based on extensive peritoneal surface disease, operating room time is not wasted on an aborted procedure.

Laparoscopy in Curative Treatment of Peritoneal Surface Malignancy

Although many complex and technically challenging procedures are now being performed in a minimally invasive fashion, laparoscopic CRS and HIPEC with curative intent remains a rare entity with few reports in the literature (**Box 4**). Laparoscopic CRS and HIPEC as curative treatment was first proposed by Esquivel and Averbach[23] after a morbidly obese woman undergoing a Roux-en-Y laparoscopic gastric bypass was intraoperatively found to have a 1-cm flat suspicious lesion on her greater omentum. This was consistent with well-differentiated papillary mesothelioma, with no other lesions on the visceral or parietal peritoneum. After a CT scan demonstrated no evidence of additional disease, she subsequently underwent laparoscopic CRS and HIPEC, including appendectomy with partial cecectomy, bilateral salpingo-oophorectomy, and omentectomy. Her PCI was 4. She had no postoperative complications and was discharged home on postoperative day 5. Follow-up imaging at 6 months showed no evidence of disease.

Box 4
Indications for laparoscopic hyperthermic intraperitoneal chemotherapy with curative intent

- Histopathologic diagnosis of peritoneal surface malignancy
- No evidence of gross peritoneal disease on computed tomography scan (estimated peritoneal cancer index of ≤10)
- Low volume peritoneal surface disease (peritoneal cancer index of ≤10) on diagnostic laparoscopy

---

Indications

With the success of their index case, Esquivel and colleagues[24] developed a protocol for laparoscopic CRS and HIPEC. Surgical candidates required a histologic diagnosis of peritoneal surface malignancy with no evidence of gross disease on CT scan. A diagnostic laparoscopy was performed, and if low volume peritoneal malignancy was identified, defined as a PCI of 10 or less, then CRS and HIPEC was continued laparoscopically. If the PCI was greater than 10 or a complete cytoreduction could not be performed laparoscopically, the procedure was converted to the standard open approach.

Passot and colleagues[25] have also developed a protocol for curative laparoscopic CRS and HIPEC in patients with low-grade appendiceal mucinous neoplasm and malignant mesothelioma. Similar to Esquivel, all patients required preoperative histologic diagnosis and abdominal imaging demonstrating minimal peritoneal surface disease (estimated PCI of ≤10). Additional criteria included American Society of Anesthesiologists (ASA) classification of 2 or less, age 75 years or younger, and a limited history of abdominal surgery (only 2 abdominal regions previously dissected). Diagnostic laparoscopy with CRS and HIPEC was performed, with planned conversion to laparotomy if the PCI became greater than 10 or disease was not amenable to complete cytoreduction by laparoscopy.

Fish and colleagues[26] also report performing laparoscopic CRS and HIPEC with a curative intent in patients with low-grade appendiceal mucinous neoplasms. All patients required a preoperative CT scan showing no peritoneal surface malignancy and only patients with no comorbidities were included. Diagnostic laparoscopy was performed and the absence of any macroscopic disease (PCI of 0) was confirmed before proceeding with prophylactic bilateral oophorectomy, omentectomy, cholecystectomy, and resection of the ligamentum teres and umbilicus followed by HIPEC.[26]

Technique

Esquivel and colleagues[24] enter the abdomen in the right upper quadrant with a 12-mm direct view visiport. After establishing a pneumoperitoneum, 2 additional 12-mm trocars are placed periumbilical and in the left upper quadrant. Two 5-mm ports are placed below the right and left costal margins, and occasionally a sixth 5-mm trocar is placed just above the pubic symphysis to facilitate upper abdomen dissection. Adhesiolysis is performed to free all intraabdominal structures and to allow for complete exploration to calculate a PCI. After exploration, if the PCI was 10 or less and all disease was amenable to laparoscopic resection, complete cytoreduction ⟍ was performed. All patients underwent greater omentectomy and bilateral salpingo-oophorectomy even if there was no evidence of macroscopic disease. When cytoreduction was complete, a 6-cm periumbilical midline incision was made to extract the specimens. Two inflow and 2 outflow cannulas were placed, and the midline incision and ports were closed at the skin to prevent leakage of chemotherapy but allow all incisions to be exposed to prevent tumor cell implantation. HIPEC was performed with cisplatin, adriamycin, or mitomycin C for 90 minutes at 43°C. After the perfusion was complete, laparoscopic trocars were reinserted and the peritoneal cavity was explored for bleeding or visceral injury. Gastrointestinal anastomoses were performed as indicated, and the midline incision and port sites were closed.

Passot and colleagues[25] described a similar technique. All patients underwent a diagnostic laparoscopy and adhesiolysis with calculation of a PCI. If the PCI was 10 or less and all disease was potentially resectable, complete CRS was undertaken. All patients underwent omentectomy regardless of the presence of macroscopic disease. HIPEC was performed using a closed abdomen technique with oxaliplatin, mitomycin C, cisplatin, or doxorubicin for 30 to 90 minutes at 42°C.

Fish and colleagues[26] described a different technique. All selected patients underwent diagnostic laparoscopy, and a laparoscopic approach was continued only if there was no macroscopic disease. Excision of the umbilicus was then performed and purse-string suture placed to close the defect around a 10-mm balloon port. In a transverse plane including the umbilical port, two 5-mm ports and two 10-mm ports were placed. A third 5-mm port was placed in the epigastric region. Using this configuration, bilateral oophorectomy, cholecystectomy, greater and lesser omentectomy, resection of the ligamentum teres, and division of the hepatophrenic ligament were performed. All specimens were placed in a bag and retrieved through the umbilical port site after release of the purse-string suture. Three patients underwent HIPEC using a modified coliseum technique using the midline umbilical incision. Seven patients had a closed technique, with inflow and outflow cannulas placed through three 12-mm laparoscopic ports placed in the right flank. All patients received Mitomycin C for 90 minutes at 41.5°C to 42.5°C. A closed suction drain was placed in the pelvis of all patients and remained for 24 hours postoperatively.

Results

Esquivel and colleagues[24] have the largest published series of laparoscopic HIPECs. In their initial series of 13 patients, 9 patients had pseudomyxoma peritonei, 1 patient had malignant mesothelioma, 2 patients had primary peritoneal surface disease, and 1 patient had colon adenocarcinoma. Three procedures were converted to open operations: the patient with colon adenocarcinoma had a PCI of greater than 10, one of the patients with primary peritoneal carcinoma's omentum could not be laparoscopically mobilized, and one patient with pseudomyxoma had a previous ileocolonic anastomosis that had tumor implants and was not amenable to laparoscopic resection. The mean PCI was 4 with a 6-day average length of stay. One grade 4 complication occurred in a patient with an internal hernia on postoperative day 7, which was reduced and repaired laparoscopically. The median follow-up time was 13 months, and all patients were disease free. In their more recent report on 19 patients with pseudomyxoma pertitonei (including 8 patients from the previous series), the mean PCI was 4.3 and the mean length of stay was 5.3 days.[27] One grade 4 complication occurred, which was the same patient in their prior published series. At mean follow-up of 17 months, all patients were disease free.

Similar results were found by Passot and colleagues,[25] who reported on 8 patients eligible for laparoscopic HIPEC, 5 with pseudomyxoma and 3 with malignant mesothelioma. No patients required conversion to open and the median PCI was 2.5. Their median length of stay was 12 days, but this was longer owing to differences in health care practices in France. At a median follow-up of 192 days, all patients were alive and disease free.

In their case series of 10 patients with pseudomyxoma peritonei, Fish and colleagues[26] reported no conversions to open procedures. A PCI of 0 was a part of their inclusion criteria. They reported a median length of stay of 7 days, and all patient were alive and disease free at a median follow-up of 3 months.

Wake Forest experience and results

At our institution, we have performed 20 laparoscopic HIPECs with curative intent between 2008 and 2017 (**Table 1**). The average age was 52 years, and 75% of patients were female. The majority of patients were Eastern Cooperative Oncology Group (ECOG) status 0 (90%), 1 patient was ECOG status 1 (5%), and 1 patient was ECOG status 2 (5%). Forty-five percent of patients were classified as ASA class 2 and 55% were ASA class 3. Appendiceal carcinoma was the most common diagnosis (85%), followed by colon cancer (10%) and mesothelioma (5%). Ninety percent of patients were perfused with mitomycin C (90%) and 10% were perfused with oxaliplatin. The majority of patients were perfused for 120 minutes (90%), but 1 patient was perfused for 60 minutes owing to poor return from the circuit and 1 patient was perfused for 105 minutes owing to a leak at the heat exchanger. The average PCI was 2, with a range from 0 to 7. All cases were R0/R1 resections. Most patients underwent at least a partial omentectomy (95%) and 35% of patients had a colectomy. No patients required an ostomy. We have found a hand port to be a valuable adjunct, because the hand port facilitates the omentectomy. Omentectomy is routinely performed with our CRS and HIPEC cases if it has not already been completed at a prior surgery. The average length of stay was 5 days, with a range of 3 to 9 days. One-half of the patients had a postoperative complication, with the majority of these being postoperative nausea. Two patients required filgastrim (Neupogen) and 1 patient had respiratory distress requiring transfer to the intensive care unit. By 30 days after laparoscopic CRS and HIPEC, 20% of patients had a complication. All complications were Clavien Dindo grade 2 or less. At 90 days postoperative, there were no complications, although the most recent case was performed in 2017 and 90 days have not elapsed. There were no deaths within 90 days. Eighty-five percent of patients are alive with no evidence of disease, 5% are alive with disease, and 10% have died. The average time to follow-up or death is 26.7 months; however, again the most recent case was performed in 2017 and less than 3 months have elapsed since her HIPEC.

Table 1
Laparoscopic hyperthermic intraperitoneal chemotherapies with curative intent

Variable	(N = 20)
Age	52.2
Sex	
Male	25%
Female	75%
Race	
White	85%
Black	10%
Hispanic	5%
ECOG	
0	90%
1	5%
2	5%
ASA	
2	45%
3	55%
Primary	
Appendix	85%
Colon	10%
Mesothelioma	5%
Grade	
Low	65%
High	35%
Mitomycin C	90%
Oxaliplatin	10%
Perfusion time	116.25
PCI	2.30
Resection	
0	30%
1	60%
Organs resected	
Diaphragm	5%
Colon	35%
Small bowel	5%
Ovaries	15%
Omentum	95%
Liver	10%
Bladder	5%
LOS	5
Complications	
In hospital	50%
30 d	20%
31–90 d	0%

(continued on next page)

Table 1 (continued)	
Variable	(N = 20)
Status	
No evidence of disease	85%
Alive with disease	5%
Dead	10%
Survival (mo)	26.7

Abbreviations: ASA, american society of anesthesiologists; ECOG, eastern cooperative oncology group; LOS, length of stay; PCI, peritoneal cancer index.

The technical aspects of laparoscopic CRS and HIPEC will vary depending on the extent of cytoreduction. Owing to the multiquadrant nature of peritoneal surface disease, there is no standard port placement configuration that is recommended. Instead, the principle of triangulation around the organ or region of the abdomen involved by peritoneal surface disease should be the guiding principle when placing laparoscopic ports.

Laparoscopic hyperthermic intraperitoneal chemotherapy as neoadjuvant or adjuvant therapy

Several studies have proposed laparoscopic HIPEC as neoadjuvant or adjuvant treatment. Chang and colleagues[28] reported the first laparoscopic HIPECs with neoadjuvant aim. Five patients with pancreatic or gastric cancer at high risk for developing peritoneal metastasis but without evidence of peritoneal dissemination underwent laparoscopic HIPEC with cisplatin and mitomycin C at the time of their laparoscopic staging. Three weeks after perfusion, they underwent open resection of their primary tumor. All 4 with patients pancreatic cancer either had recurrent disease or died; the patient with gastric cancer was alive at 43 months with no evidence of disease. Several Japanese groups are performing laparoscopic HIPEC in the neoadjuvant setting followed by interval gastrectomy for patients with gastric cancer metastases limited to the peritoneum, and suggest there may be a benefit.[29,30] Badgwell and colleagues[31] at MD Anderson Cancer Center conducted a phase II trial in patients with gastric cancer with peritoneal metastases where patients underwent at least 1 laparoscopic HIPEC after completing systemic chemotherapy. Patients with negative peritoneal washings and no evidence of peritoneal disease were offered gastrectomy. Of 19 patients enrolled, however, only 5 had negative washings and went on to resection.

Laparoscopic HIPEC has also been suggested as a staged procedure performed several weeks after open CRS owing to concern that HIPEC immediately after CRS may contribute to the high complication rate. Knutsen and colleagues[32] performed 5 staged laparoscopic HIPECs on patients with peritoneal surface disease from appendiceal, gallbladder, and small bowel adenocarcinoma. Four patients had no complications from the laparoscopic HIPEC and 1 patient's course was complicated by cellulitis. The patient with small bowel disease died less than 1 year after treatment. The other 4 patients had no evidence of disease at 1 year of follow-up.

Although laparoscopic HIPEC as a neoadjuvant or adjuvant modality has been proposed, we do not recommend this because of a lack of data on its effectiveness. All of the reports in the literature have been small case series with varying efficacy and results. Although laparoscopic HIPEC seems to be safe with low morbidity in the neoadjuvant or adjuvant setting, further studies are warranted.

Laparoscopy in Palliative Treatment of Malignant Ascites

Indications and results

Malignant ascites is one of the most common comorbid conditions accompanying peritoneal surface disease and can occur with a wide range of neoplasms, including ovarian cancer, colon cancer, stomach cancer, breast cancer, melanoma, and mesothelioma.[33,34] Loss of proteins and electrolyte disorders can cause diffuse edema, and the accumulation of fluid can facilitate sepsis, all contributing to a significant loss in patient quality of life.[35] Treatment options include diuretics, paracentesis, immunotherapy, and shunts, all with varying, but limited, degrees of efficacy and morbidity (**Box 5**).

Box 5
Indications for palliative laparoscopic hyperthermic intraperitoneal chemotherapy for malignant ascites

- Peritoneal surface disease not amenable to complete cytoreduction
- Refractory ascites after other treatment modalities
- Highly symptomatic with decreased quality of life

HIPEC has been proposed as a treatment strategy for patients who have refractory malignant ascites and who are not candidates for curative CRS.[34,36] Our institution examined the efficacy of HIPEC in controlling malignant ascites in patients in whom complete CRS was attempted but was not completed as a result of the distribution or volume of disease.[36] Malignant ascites was found in 299 patients who underwent 310 procedures. The majority of the patients had an appendiceal primary (46%), followed by colorectal cancer (17%), and mesothelioma (15%). Most patients underwent a 120-minute perfusion (78%) with mitomycin C (83%). Complete resolution of malignant ascites occurred in 93% of the cases, and 84% of these still had residual macroscopic disease (R2 resection). In the 7% of cases where the ascites did not completely resolve, the majority (86%) were R2 resections. There was no statistically significant difference in resolution of ascites based on resection status, primary tumor, perfusion duration, or perfusion agent. This finding suggested that the resolution of malignant ascites is more likely a function of HIPEC rather than CRS.

Laparoscopic HIPEC has been suggested as a less invasive method for HIPEC in patients with known malignant ascites who are not candidates for curative CRS based on preoperative imaging.[34,36] These patients are highly symptomatic and have refractory ascites despite treatment with other less aggressive modalities. Multiple series have demonstrated the efficacy and safety of laparoscopic palliative HIPEC in a wide range of tumor types. Valle and colleagues[34] performed laparoscopic HIPEC in 52 patients with debilitating malignant ascites who had undergone previous conventional treatment without symptom relief. The most common primary malignancy treated was gastric adenocarcinoma, followed by colon cancer, ovarian cancer, breast cancer, peritoneal mesothelioma, and melanoma. One month after laparoscopic HIPEC, CT scanning demonstrated complete resolution of ascites in 49 of 52 patients (94%), with 2 of the 3 recurrences considered small and clinically irrelevant. One patient was symptomatic again at 3 months and received a second laparoscopic HIPEC with complete resolution of ascites on follow-up imaging. Postoperative complications included 2 wound infections and 1 deep vein thrombosis. Importantly, the Karnofsky performance status improved by an average of 20 points in the postoperative period.

There are several other reports in the literature of complete resolution of malignant ascites after laparoscopic HIPEC. Facchiano and colleagues[37] performed laparoscopic HIPEC on 5 patients with peritoneal metastases from gastric cancer, and all patients had complete resolution of their ascites with no related morbidity or mortality. Garofalo and Valle[20] found similar results in 14 patients with gastric cancer, colon cancer, ovarian cancer, breast cancer, and mesothelioma peritoneal surface disease, demonstrating complete resolution of ascites in all patients. Ba and colleagues[38] performed continuous laparoscopic HIPEC on 16 patients with ascites from gastric adenocarcinoma. The first session was completed in the operating room and perfusion catheters were left in place. Two additional perfusions were performed in the intensive care unit on the first and second days after the operation. Clinically complete resolution of ascites was achieved in 14 patients (90.5%), and partial resolution in 2 patients (9.5%). Karnofsky scores increased in all patients, with a significant difference before and after treatment.

Laparoscopic evacuation of mucinous ascites without HIPEC has also been proposed as a palliative strategy.[39] Kelly and colleagues[39] described 10 patients with pseudomyxoma peritonei who underwent laparoscopy with evacuation of mucin. Eight patients had low-grade disease and 2 patients had high-grade disease. Two patients underwent multiple repeat procedures, with 1 patient undergoing 5 procedures in a 15-month period and the other undergoing 4 procedures over 5 years. The median volume of mucin evacuated was 2.0 L, with a range of 1.7 to 8.0 L. Frequent bed tilting with inspection of all 4 quadrants and irrigation with sterile saline to reduce the viscosity of the mucin were used to facilitate complete evacuation. All patients reported significant improvement in bloating and early satiety. The only complication was one patient with persistent leakage from a port site. Median time to recurrence of symptoms was 5.3 months, with a median follow-up of 9.1 months. There were 2 deaths owing to disease, both of whom had high-grade histology. Based on this small series, Kelly and colleagues[39] suggest that, for patients with pseudomyxoma peritonei in whom distension is the primary symptom requiring palliation, selection criteria for laparoscopic evacuation should include (1) large volume mucinous ascites ($\geq$1 L), (2) mucinous ascites accessible without intervening bowel, (3) medically fit enough for laparotomy should conversion to open be necessary, and (4) a life expectancy of 6 months or longer.

Malignant ascites is a highly morbid condition found in many end-stage cancers. Although there are several conventional treatments that provide symptom relief, they are often only temporary or carry their own associated morbidity. Using laparoscopic HIPEC to achieve complete, lasting resolution of malignant ascites has been shown to be both safe and effective for a wide range of primary malignancies. The approach to laparoscopic HIPEC for malignant ascites has not yet been standardized and still relies heavily on appropriate patient selection and surgeon familiarity; however, with increasing experience laparoscopic HIPEC is becoming an attractive option for patients with refractory malignant ascites.

SUMMARY

Treatment strategies for patients with peritoneal surface malignancies have significantly evolved in the last 30 years. Patients who would traditionally have been considered to have end-stage disease are now undergoing CRS and HIPEC with curative intent. Increasingly complex procedures are now being performed laparoscopically, and laparoscopic CRS and HIPEC has been shown to be a viable option in carefully selected patients. We advocate for laparoscopic HIPEC with curative intent in patients with low volume disease (PCI of ≤10) on preoperative imaging or initial diagnostic laparoscopy whose tumor burden would be amenable to complete laparoscopic CRS. Laparoscopic HIPEC has also been shown to be effective in patients with intractable malignant ascites who are not candidates for complete cytoreduction and have debilitating symptoms. Continued study and clinical trials of these promising treatment strategies for peritoneal surface malignancy as they continue to advance are warranted.

REFERENCES

1. Sugarbaker PH, Chang D. Results of treatment of 385 patients with peritoneal surface spread of appendiceal malignancy. Ann Surg Oncol 1999;6(8):727–31.
2. Glehen O, Kwiatkowski F, Sugarbaker PH, et al. Cytoreductive surgery combined with perioperative intraperitoneal chemotherapy for the management of peritoneal carcinomatosis from colorectal cancer: a multi-institutional study. J Clin Oncol 2004;22(16):3284–92.
3. Glehen O, Schreiber V, Cotte E, et al. Cytoreductive surgery and intraperitoneal chemohyperthermia for peritoneal carcinomatosis arising from gastric cancer. Arch Surg 2004;139(1):20–6.
4. Feldman AL, Libutti SK, Pingpank JF, et al. Analysis of factors associated with outcome in patients with malignant peritoneal mesothelioma undergoing surgical debulking and intraperitoneal chemotherapy. J Clin Oncol 2003;21(24):4560–7.
5. Verwaal VJ, van Ruth S, de Bree E, et al. Randomized trial of cytoreduction and hyperthermic intraperitoneal chemotherapy versus systemic chemotherapy and palliative surgery in patients with peritoneal carcinomatosis of colorectal cancer. J Clin Oncol 2003;21(20):3737–43.
6. Chua TC, Robertson G, Liauw W, et al. Intraoperative hyperthermic intraperitoneal chemotherapy after cytoreductive surgery in ovarian cancer peritoneal carcinomatosis: systematic review of current results. J Cancer Res Clin Oncol 2009;135(12):1637–45.
7. van Driel WJ, Koole SN, Sikorska K, et al. Hyperthermic intraperitoneal chemotherapy in ovarian cancer. N Engl J Med 2018;378(3):230–40.
8. Chua TC, Yan TD, Saxena A, et al. Should the treatment of peritoneal carcinomatosis by cytoreductive surgery and hyperthermic intraperitoneal chemotherapy still be regarded as a highly morbid procedure? A systematic review of morbidity and mortality. Ann Surg 2009;249(6):900–7.
9. Ceelen WP, Levine EA. Intraperitoneal cancer therapy: principles and practice.
10. Verwaal VJ, Kusamura S, Baratti D, et al. The eligibility for local-regional treatment of peritoneal surface malignancy. J Surg Oncol 2008;98(4):220–3.
11. Valle M, Federici O, Garofalo A. Patient selection for cytoreductive surgery and hyperthermic intraperitoneal chemotherapy, and role of laparoscopy in diagnosis, staging, and treatment. Surg Oncol Clin N Am 2012;21(4):515–31.
12. Jacquet P, Jelinek JS, Steves MA, et al. Evaluation of computed tomography in patients with peritoneal carcinomatosis. Cancer 1993;72(5):1631–6.
13. Edge SB, American Joint Committee on Cancer, American Cancer Society. AJCC cancer staging handbook: from the AJCC cancer staging manual. 7th edition. New York: Springer; 2010.
14. Glehen O, Mithieux F, Osinsky D, et al. Surgery combined with peritonectomy procedures and intraperitoneal chemohyperthermia in abdominal cancers with peritoneal carcinomatosis: a phase II study. J Clin Oncol 2003;21(5):799–806.

15. Sugarbaker PH, Jablonski KA. Prognostic features of 51 colorectal and 130 appendiceal cancer patients with peritoneal carcinomatosis treated by cytoreductive surgery and intraperitoneal chemotherapy. Ann Surg 1995;221(2):124–32.

16. Elias D, Blot F, El Otmany A, et al. Curative treatment of peritoneal carcinomatosis arising from colorectal cancer by complete resection and intraperitoneal chemotherapy. Cancer 2001;92(1):71–6.

17. Yonemura Y, Fujimura T, Nishimura G, et al. Effects of intraoperative chemohyperthermia in patients with gastric cancer with peritoneal dissemination. Surgery 1996;119(4):437–44.

18. Harmon RL, Sugarbaker PH. Prognostic indicators in peritoneal carcinomatosis from gastrointestinal cancer. Int Semin Surg Oncol 2005;2(1):3.

19. Denzer U, Hoffmann S, Helmreich-Becker I, et al. Minilaparoscopy in the diagnosis of peritoneal tumor spread: prospective controlled comparison with computed tomography. Surg Endosc 2004;18(7):1067–70.

20. Garofalo A, Valle M. Laparoscopy in the management of peritoneal carcinomatosis. Cancer J 2009;15(3):190–5.

21. Valle M, Garofalo A. Laparoscopic staging of peritoneal surface malignancies. Eur J Surg Oncol 2006;32(6):625–7.

22. Hirano M, Yonemura Y, Canbay E, et al. Laparoscopic diagnosis and laparoscopic hyperthermic intraoperative intraperitoneal chemotherapy for pseudomyxoma peritonei detected by CT examination. Gastroenterol Res Pract 2012;2012: 741202.

23. Esquivel J, Averbach A. Combined laparoscopic cytoreductive surgery and hyperthermic intraperitoneal chemotherapy in a patient with peritoneal mesothelioma. J Laparoendosc Adv Surg Tech A 2009;19(4):505–7.

24. Esquivel J, Averbach A, Chua TC. Laparoscopic cytoreductive surgery and hyperthermic intraperitoneal chemotherapy in patients with limited peritoneal surface malignancies: feasibility, morbidity and outcome in an early experience. Ann Surg 2011;253(4):764–8.

25. Passot G, Bakrin N, Isaac S, et al. Postoperative outcomes of laparoscopic vs open cytoreductive surgery plus hyperthermic intraperitoneal chemotherapy for treatment of peritoneal surface malignancies. Eur J Surg Oncol 2014;40(8): 957–62.

26. Fish R, Selvasekar C, Crichton P, et al. Risk-reducing laparoscopic cytoreductive surgery and hyperthermic intraperitoneal chemotherapy for low-grade appendiceal mucinous neoplasm: early outcomes and technique. Surg Endosc 2014; 28(1):341–5.

27. Esquivel J, Averbach A. Laparoscopic cytoreductive surgery and HIPEC in patients with limited pseudomyxoma peritonei of appendiceal origin. Gastroenterol Res Pract 2012;2012:981245.

28. Chang E, Alexander HR, Libutti SK, et al. Laparoscopic continuous hyperthermic peritoneal perfusion. J Am Coll Surg 2001;193(2):225–9.

29. Yonemura Y, Canbay E, Sako S, et al. Effects of laparoscopic hyperthermic intraperitoneal chemotherapy for peritoneal metastasis from gastric cancer. Canc Clin Oncol 2014;3(2):43–50.

30. Yan TD, Black D, Sugarbaker PH, et al. A systematic review and meta-analysis of the randomized controlled trials on adjuvant intraperitoneal chemotherapy for resectable gastric cancer. Ann Surg Oncol 2007;14(10):2702–13.

31. Badgwell B, Blum M, Das P, et al. Phase II trial of laparoscopic hyperthermic intraperitoneal chemoperfusion for peritoneal carcinomatosis or positive

peritoneal cytology in patients with gastric adenocarcinoma. Ann Surg Oncol 2017;24(11):3338–44.

32. Knutsen A, Sielaff TD, Greeno E, et al. Staged laparoscopic infusion of hyperthermic intraperitoneal chemotherapy after cytoreductive surgery. J Gastrointest Surg 2006;10(7):1038–43.

33. Facchiano E, Risio D, Kianmanesh R, et al. Laparoscopic hyperthermic intraperitoneal chemotherapy: indications, aims, and results: a systematic review of the literature. Ann Surg Oncol 2012;19(9):2946–50.

34. Valle M, Van der Speeten K, Garofalo A. Laparoscopic hyperthermic intraperitoneal peroperative chemotherapy (HIPEC) in the management of refractory malignant ascites: a multi-institutional retrospective analysis in 52 patients. J Surg Oncol 2009;100(4):331–4.

35. Cavazzoni E, Bugiantella W, Graziosi L, et al. Malignant ascites: pathophysiology and treatment. Int J Clin Oncol 2013;18(1):1–9.

36. Randle RW, Swett KR, Swords DS, et al. Efficacy of cytoreductive surgery with hyperthermic intraperitoneal chemotherapy in the management of malignant ascites. Ann Surg Oncol 2014;21(5):1474–9.

37. Facchiano E, Scaringi S, Kianmanesh R, et al. Laparoscopic hyperthermic intraperitoneal chemotherapy (HIPEC) for the treatment of malignant ascites secondary to unresectable peritoneal carcinomatosis from advanced gastric cancer. Eur J Surg Oncol 2008;34(2):154–8.

38. Ba MC, Cui SZ, Lin SQ, et al. Chemotherapy with laparoscope-assisted continuous circulatory hyperthermic intraperitoneal perfusion for malignant ascites. World J Gastroenterol 2010;16(15):1901–7.

39. Kelly KJ, Baumgartner JM, Lowy AM. Laparoscopic evacuation of mucinous ascites for palliation of pseudomyxoma peritonei. Ann Surg Oncol 2015;22(5):1722–5.

Minimally Invasive Esophageal Cancer Surgery

June S. Peng, MD, Moshim Kukar, MD, Gary N. Mann, MD,
Steven N. Hochwald, MD, MBA*

KEYWORDS

- Esophageal cancer • Gastroesophageal junction cancer • Neoadjuvant therapy
- Minimally invasive esophagectomy
- Robotic-assisted minimally invasive esophagectomy

KEY POINTS

- Minimally invasive esophagectomy can be performed for most oncologic resections with the benefit of decreased complications and faster recovery.
- Selection between minimally invasive Ivor Lewis, McKeown, and transhiatal esophagectomy depends on tumor and patient characteristics.
- The steps of laparoscopic and robotic Ivor Lewis, McKeown, and transhiatal esophagectomy are described within this article.
- Postoperative management of patients after minimally invasive esophagectomy should follow a clinical pathway to expedite recovery and minimize complications.

INTRODUCTION

The incidence of esophageal cancer in the United States for 2018 is estimated to be 17,290 cases, with 15,850 deaths.[1] Globally, esophageal cancer is the eighth most common cancer and the sixth leading cause of cancer death.[2] The financial cost of treating esophageal cancer is one of the highest among common cancers.[3]

Squamous cell carcinoma (SCC) is most common worldwide, with the highest incidence in Asia, Africa, and South America.[2] These tumors are more likely to be in the proximal and mid esophagus, with greater likelihood of being unresectable because of local invasion of critical structures such as the trachea. Adenocarcinoma (AC) is more common in the United States and Western countries, arising in the distal esophageal and gastroesophageal junction (GEJ), commonly with involvement of a limited amount of stomach and frequent involvement of intra-abdominal lymph nodes.

Disclosures: The authors have no disclosures.
Department of Surgical Oncology, Roswell Park Comprehensive Cancer Center, 665 Elm Street, Buffalo, NY 14203, USA
* Corresponding author. Department of Surgical Oncology, Clinical Sciences Center P-637, Roswell Park Comprehensive Cancer Center, 665 Elm Street, Buffalo, NY 14203.
E-mail address: steven.hochwald@roswellpark.org

Surg Oncol Clin N Am 28 (2019) 177–200
https://doi.org/10.1016/j.soc.2018.11.009
1055-3207/19/© 2018 Elsevier Inc. All rights reserved.

surgonc.theclinics.com

NEOADJUVANT THERAPY

In general, patients with T1a tumors are referred for endoscopic mucosal resection or endoscopic submucosal dissection, and fit patients with T1b tumors are most appropriate for upfront esophagectomy. Patients with T2-T4 tumors and/or nodal disease are referred for neoadjuvant chemoradiation based on improved pathologic and survival outcomes demonstrated in randomized trials.

The CROSS trial (ChemoRadiotherapy for Oesophageal cancer follow by Surgery Study) randomized 368 patients with esophageal or GEJ cancer to neoadjuvant carboplatin and paclitaxel with concurrent radiation followed by surgery versus surgery alone.[4] The neoadjuvant group had more margin negative resections (92 vs 69%, $P = .001$) with complete pathologic response in 23% of AC and 49% of SCC, and improved median overall survival (49.4 months vs 24.0 months, $P = .003$). Perioperative chemotherapy for patients with GEJ tumors has also been shown to be beneficial. The MAGIC trial (Medical Research Council Adjuvant Gastric Infusional Chemotherapy) randomized 503 patients with gastric, GEJ, and lower esophageal cancer to perioperative epirubicin, cisplatin, and fluorouracil (ECF) and surgery versus surgery alone. Overall survival at 5 years in the perioperative chemotherapy group was 36% versus 23% for surgery alone ($P = .009$).[5] More recently, the FLOT4-AIO (Arbeitsgemeinschaft Internistische Onkologie) trial reported superiority of perioperative FLOT (fluorouracil, leucovorin, oxaliplatin, and docetaxel) with median overall survival of 50 months compared with 35 months with ECF ($P = .012$).[6] Limitations of the MAGIC and FLOT4 trials for patients with GEJ cancer are that only a minority of patients in both trials had tumors located at the GEJ, whereas most patients had gastric involvement only.

The nutritional status of the patient should be evaluated with attention during history and physical examination to degree of dysphagia and weight loss. Feeding jejunostomy should be placed before neoadjuvant therapy in patients with difficulty maintaining oral intake or demonstrating significant malnutrition. Smoking and alcohol cessation resources should be provided for relevant patients.

Patients are restaged 4 weeks after completion of neoadjuvant therapy with PET-computed tomography (CT), and those without evidence of metastatic disease undergo esophagectomy 6 to 10 weeks after completion of neoadjuvant therapy. Pulmonary function and cardiac testing are performed as clinically indicated.

SURGICAL APPROACH

The goals of esophagectomy are oncologic resection with negative margins and adequate lymphadenectomy.[7] The choice of approach depends on the experience of the surgeon and the anatomy of the patient. In the authors' experience, almost all patients can be considered for minimally invasive esophagectomy (MIE), with decreased complication rates and faster recovery. A recent review of the National Cancer Database demonstrated a temporal increase in MIEs with 55.9% of esophagectomies performed laparoscopically or robotically in 2015.[8]

Two randomized trials have compared minimally invasive to open esophagectomy. The TIME trial (Traditional Invasive vs Minimally invasive Esophagectomy) randomized 115 patients to open esophagectomy with laparotomy and thoracotomy or MIE with laparoscopy and thoracoscopy, with thoracic or neck anastomoses in both groups.[9] The MIE group had significantly lower rates of pulmonary infection (9% vs 29%, $P = .005$), with no difference in margin status, nodal yield, or mortality. In addition, secondary endpoints included 3 quality-of-life measurements, which were all significantly improved in the MIE group. Finally, length of hospital stay was significantly shorter in the MIE group. A recent update from this trial showed no difference in 3-year disease-free or overall survival.[10] The ROBOT trial (Robot-assisted Thoracolaparoscopic Esophagectomy vs Open Transthoracic Esophagectomy) was reported in abstract form and randomized 112 patients to robotic-assisted MIE (RAMIE) or open esophagectomy.[11] The RAMIE group had fewer Clavien-Dindo grade 2 and more severe complications (59 vs 80%, $P = .02$) and less surgical, pulmonary, and cardiac complications. Pathologic and oncologic survival outcomes were equivalent. Therefore, both randomized trials that have been reported to date, comparing MIE to open esophagectomy, support the routine use of minimally invasive approaches for esophageal and GEJ cancer.

The 3 commonly used approaches for MIE are McKeown or 3-field, Ivor Lewis (IL-MIE), and transhiatal or transmediastinal (TH-MIE). The stomach is preferred as the conduit for restoration of intestinal tract continuity in all approaches.

A McKeown esophagectomy requires dissection in the abdomen, right thorax, and neck, with a cervical anastomosis. The authors use this approach for patients with midesophageal or more proximal tumors or significant regional nodal disease and need for 3 field lymph node dissection. This approach is avoided, if possible, in patients with a history of neck surgery or irradiation, or prior gastric surgery, which may compromise gastric conduit length. Because the anastomosis is in the neck, the operation requires less time in the chest, which may benefit patients with underlying pulmonary disease. McKeown esophagectomy is associated with a higher rate of recurrent laryngeal nerve (RLN) injury[12] and higher leak rate.[13] The largest single-institution series of 481 McKeown MIEs reported anastomotic leaks requiring reoperation in 5.4%, vocal cord paralysis in 7.7%, and 30-day mortality of 2.5%.[12] Another series of 247 McKeown MIEs reported a leak rate of 8.5% with a very low rate of reoperation for leaks.[14] The oncologic outcomes of McKeown MIE are comparable to open esophagectomy, with Luketich and colleagues[12] reporting a negative margin in 98% and median nodal yield of 19. Another institutional series of 108 patients confirmed adequate pathologic and oncologic outcomes with a 95% margin negative resection rate, median lymph node yield of 26, and 5-year overall survival of 42%.[15]

An Ivor Lewis esophagectomy is the authors' preferred approach for an MIE and requires abdominal and right thoracic dissection with an intrathoracic anastomosis. Luketich and colleagues[12] reported 530 IL-MIEs with anastomotic leaks requiring reoperation in 4.3%, vocal cord paresis in 0.9%, and 30-day mortality of 0.9%. The margin negative rate was 98%, and median nodal yield was 23.5. The authors' experience likewise showed a leak rate of 4.4% for IL-MIE and that reoperation for leaks was rarely necessary.[14] A multi-institutional review compared 356 patients who underwent MIE with thoracic or cervical anastomosis and showed that thoracic anastomosis was associated with a lower rate of RLN palsy (0 vs 14.4%, $P<.001$), strictures requiring dilation (6.2% vs 42.8%, $P<.001$), and better functional results.[16] These institutional series suggest a benefit to intrathoracic anastomosis, and there is currently a randomized trial in progress comparing cervical versus thoracic anastomosis.[17]

Transhiatal or transmediastinal esophagectomy involves dissection of the esophagus from the abdomen and neck, without entering the chest. The authors consider this approach in patients with relatively poor pulmonary function or active smoking in whom single lung ventilation would be poorly tolerated, or patients with a history of significant right lung surgery. This approach is relatively contraindicated if there is bulky mediastinal disease and can be challenging in patients with morbid obesity or cardiomegaly. The largest series reported 72 patients who underwent TH-MIE with a leak rate of 19%, median nodal yield of 11, and margin negative resection in all patients.[18] Another series of 40 patients reported median lymph node yield of 20, margin negative resection in 94.7%, but also high complication rates with anastomotic leak in 25% and RLN paresis in 35%.[19] A systematic review of published series of TH-MIE and TH-RAMIE included 8 series encompassing 334 patients and reported anastomotic leak rates of 3% to 29%, in-hospital mortality of 0% to 6%, margin negative resection in 74% to 100%, and median nodal yield of 3 to 20.[20]

The learning curves for MIE and RAMIE are substantial and require investment in personnel, equipment, and resources for success. Both approaches confer benefits compared with open esophagectomy and the choice between laparoscopic or robotic MIE and which of the 3 approaches (IL, TH, or McKeown) depends on surgeon training and local resources. The learning curve to transition from open to IL-MIE was reported at 119 cases based on an analysis of leak rates in 646 patients.[21] The transition from open to RAMIE in a single surgeon series, which included McKeown and IL-RAMIE, reported that vocal cord palsy peaked at 60 cases, operative time peaked at 80 cases, and anastomotic leak peaked at 86 cases.[22] For surgeons facile in laparoscopic esophagectomy, there is an additional learning curve of 26 cases to transition to McKeown RAMIE[23] with similar curve expected for the other approaches.

SURGICAL TECHNIQUE
Operative Sequence

McKeown: Start in left lateral decubitus position for thoracic dissection, then supine for the neck and abdominal portions.

Ivor Lewis: Start supine for abdominal dissection, then left lateral decubitus.

Transhiatal: Supine throughout.

Anesthesia and Preoperative Considerations

In the preoperative holding area, patients receive prophylactic subcutaneous heparin, and acetaminophen, gabapentin, and celecoxib as part of an enhanced recovery after surgery pathway protocol.

Patients undergo general anesthesia with placement of a double-lumen endotracheal tube or single-lumen tube with a bronchial blocker for lung isolation. Bronchoscopy is performed to confirm appropriate positioning of the tube after insertion and after the patient is repositioned.

Central venous access is rarely required. An arterial line is placed and used with the Vigileo system (Edwards Lifesciences, Irvine, CA, USA) for hemodynamic monitoring. Intraoperative fluid administration is minimized, starting at a maintenance rate of 75 mL per hour with adjustments based on hemodynamic parameters and stroke volume variation.

An 18-French nasogastric tube (NGT) and Foley catheter are placed. Antibiotic prophylaxis is administered per institutional guidelines.

Abdominal Operation: Laparoscopic

Positioning

The patient is positioned supine with footboard in place. The left arm is tucked for McKeown or TH-MIE. For IL-MIE, a beanbag is placed to facilitate positioning for the subsequent thoracic dissection. For McKeown or TH-MIE, a bump is placed under the scapulae; the neck is extended, and the patient's head is slightly rotated to the right. The skin preparation should encompass the neck, chest, and abdomen into one field.

Port placement

Three 5-mm ports and one 12-mm or 15-mm port are placed (**Fig. 1**), approximately 18 to 20 cm inferior to the xiphoid process and a hand's width apart, with the jejunostomy tube site reserved in the left abdomen.

Instruments

The authors use long instruments (45 cm), including Debakey graspers on Snowden-Pencer in-line handles (Becton, Dickinson and Company, Franklin Lakes, NJ, USA), 45-cm Enseal tissue sealer (Ethicon, Somerville, NJ, USA), Endo Stitch suturing device (Medtronic, Minneapolis, MN, USA), 5-mm automatic titanium clip-applier, Endo GIA stapler (Medtronic), 0° and 30° 5-mm laparoscopes with high-definition cameras (Karl Storz, Germany).

Operation

The operating surgeon stands on the patient's right, and the assistant stands on the left. The abdominal cavity is entered with a direct optical view port entry in the left upper quadrant.

The peritoneal cavity is examined for metastatic disease.

A Nathanson liver retractor is placed, and the patient is positioned into steep reverse Trendelenburg position.

The pars flaccida is opened toward the right crus, and a retrogastric tunnel is created at the hiatus. A thin (1/4-inch) Penrose drain is passed and secured with an Endoloop (Ethicon) for retraction.

The greater curve dissection begins with division of the gastrocolic ligament with entry into the lesser sac (**Fig. 2**). Traction is provided by grasping the stomach itself, avoiding manipulation of the gastroepiploic vessels. Dissection is carried out with the Enseal, and the left gastroepiploic, posterior, and short gastric vessels are divided until the left crus is visualized. To accomplish this dissection, the surgeon's left hand grasps the posterior gastric wall while flipping the gastroepiploic vessels anteriorly. A

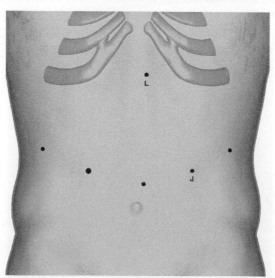

Fig. 1. Laparoscopic port placement for abdominal dissection and conduit creation, with jejunostomy tube (J) and liver retractor (L) sites indicated. (*Adapted from* BodyParts3D, licensed under CC Attribution-Share Alike 2.1 Japan. Available at: https://creativecommons.org/licenses/by-sa/2.1/jp/deed.en_US.)

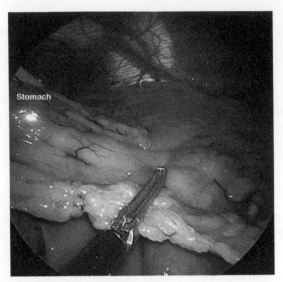

Fig. 2. Laparoscopic greater curve dissection.

6- to 7-cm portion of omentum near the inferior pole of the spleen is kept with the stomach, which will be used later to cover the anastomosis. A much larger pedicle of omentum is left on the stomach wall for IL-MIE.

To mobilize the lower portion of the stomach, the gastropancreatic folds are divided with cautery, and the gastrocolic ligament is opened distally by retracting the antrum toward the GEJ. The transverse mesocolon is dissected from the gastroepiploic bundle by the assistant (**Fig. 3**), proceeding until the gastroduodenal artery (GDA) is exposed. It is important to identify the GDA early in the dissection so that the origin of the right gastroepiploic vessels can be identified and preserved.

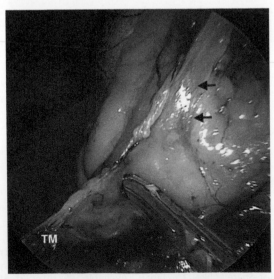

Fig. 3. Transverse mesocolon (TM) dissection from the gastroepiploic pedicle (*arrows*).

The duodenum is mobilized until the bile duct is visualized and the pylorus can reach the hiatus without tension. A formal Kocher maneuver is typically not required.

The right gastric artery is dissected on the lesser curvature of the gastric wall approximately 4 cm proximal to the pylorus and divided with the Enseal (**Fig. 4**).

The left gastric and celiac axis lymphadenectomy is performed by opening the retroperitoneum on the superior border of the pancreas and sweeping the nodal tissue up with the specimen (**Fig. 5**). The left gastric vein is clipped or divided with the Enseal. The left gastric artery is skeletonized using hook cautery, keeping the nodal tissue with the specimen, and divided with a vascular load stapler. The proximal splenic artery is also cleared of nodal disease.

The retrogastric dissection is completed; the phrenoesophageal ligament is divided, and the GEJ is mobilized widely, dissecting the left and right crura away from the esophagus. Any hiatal hernia is reduced into the abdominal cavity.

The NGT is pulled back by the anesthesia team. The conduit is created using 60-mm Endo GIA loads with 4.8-mm staple height, starting on the lesser curve 4 cm proximal to the pylorus. Reinforced staple loads are used for IL-MIE (**Fig. 6**), while unreinforced loads are used if the gastric conduit is to be pulled up to the neck. The first fire typically requires a 3- to 4-cm bite with full articulation of the stapler into the gastric lumen to narrow the conduit. The tubularized conduit should be approximately 5 to 6 cm wide. Bleeding from the staple lines can be controlled with a simple interrupted silk stitch.

Following creation of the gastric conduit and division of the stomach, the dissection of the esophagus is extended into the lower mediastinum, taking care to include the paracardial lymph nodes with the specimen and avoiding entry into the left pleural space for IL or McKeown MIE, and avoiding both pleural spaces for TH-MIE. The Penrose drain is pushed into the mediastinum and left for later retrieval during the thoracic portion of the case if performing an IL-MIE.

For TH-MIE, dissection proceeds into the mediastinum, with frequent readjustment of tension to permit circumferential dissection of the esophagus. Care should be taken to avoid injury to the membranous portion of the trachea and the azygous vein anteriorly, and the aorta posteriorly. Posterior vascular and lymphatic branches along the

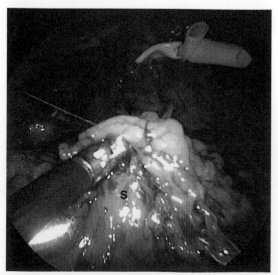

Fig. 4. Laparoscopic right gastric artery (*arrow*) dissection from the stomach (S) wall.

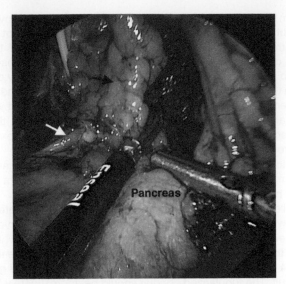

Fig. 5. Laparoscopic celiac axis and left gastric pedicle lymphadenectomy. The left gastric vein (*white arrow*) and left gastric pedicle (*black arrow*) are visible.

right side of the esophagus should be clipped to avoid injury to the thoracic duct and then divided using the Enseal. The vagus nerves are divided. Dissection proceeds superiorly, avoiding incursion into the pleural spaces, and circumferential dissection continues until the esophagus is mobilized about two-thirds of the way up to the neck. At this point, a cervical incision is made, and cervical dissection proceeds as described later. Dissection then continues from the transhiatal approach and alternates with the cervical approach until the esophagus is fully mobilized up to the cervical region. Finally, the tip of the gastric conduit is attached to the specimen using 2 interrupted 2-0 silk stitches.

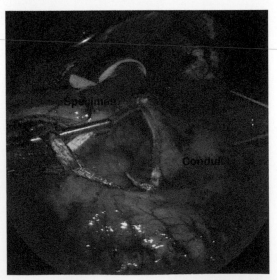

Fig. 6. Laparoscopic gastric conduit creation with reinforced staple loads.

For McKeown and TH-MIE, the specimen and conduit are gently pulled up to the neck by the assistant standing on the left.[24] The surgeon on the right side of the table assists by guiding and orienting the conduit to prevent twisting. Three to 4 long sutures are placed on the lesser curvature side of the conduit, to reinforce the staple line and serve as handles to assist with conduit positioning. The cervical anastomosis is performed, and then the esophagus and stomach are returned to the mediastinum. The conduit is pulled gently back into the abdomen to avoid redundant conduit in the mediastinum, which can lead to emptying issues. The conduit is tacked to the left diaphragm to prevent herniation of intra-abdominal contents.

The authors routinely inject the pyloric ring anteriorly and posteriorly with 50 to 100 units of botulinum toxin (Allergan, Dublin, Ireland) dissolved in 10 mL of saline, rather than performing a pyloroplasty.

A modified 16-French T-tube is routinely placed as a feeding jejunostomy, with the technique described previously.[25]

The 12-mm or 15-mm port site is closed, and port sites are injected with a long-acting local anesthetic. No drains are used for the abdominal portion of the case. Chest tubes are placed if the pleural spaces were widely opened during TH-MIE. Skin is closed and dressed with Dermabond skin adhesive (Ethicon), which can be prepared during the thoracic portion of the case.

Abdominal Operation: Robotic

Positioning

The patient is positioned supine, with arms tucked, and footboard in place, and with the table rotated slightly clockwise. The authors use a Pink Pad (Xodus Medical, Pittsburgh, PA, USA) for RAMIEs to provide padding and grip. For McKeown or TH-MIE, a bump is placed under the scapulae, and the patient's head is rotated to the right.

Port placement

The authors use the Da Vinci Xi robotic platform (Intuitive Surgical, Sunnyvale, CA, USA) docked from the patient's left side. Three 8-mm robotic, one 12-mm robotic, and one 5-mm assistant ports are placed (**Fig. 7**). These ports are 8 to 10 cm apart at the level of the umbilicus for McKeown or IL-MIE, and 2 to 3 cm higher for TH-MIE in order to reach the upper mediastinum. The assistant port is inferior and between arms 2 and 3 of the robot. A 12-mm assistant port can be used instead of a 5-mm port to expedite introduction of sutures later in the case. The authors find use of the AirSeal insufflation system (CONMED, Utica, NY, USA) helpful only for TH-MIE. A Nathanson liver retractor is placed in the subxiphoid location, with the arm positioned low to the bed to avoid collision with the robotic arms.

Instruments

Instruments used include an atraumatic grasper, such as Cadiere, fenestrated bipolar, hook or scissors, vessel sealer, 30° scope, 0° scope for TH-MIE, and a robotic stapler.

Operation

The overall steps and technique for RAMIE are similar to MIE. The deviations and robotic-specific considerations are outlined. Of note, robotic ports are placed a few centimeters inferiorly compared with laparoscopic ports.

The 30° robotic camera is placed in arm 3.

The greater curve mobilization and dissection of the transverse mesocolon from the gastroepiploic bundle are performed with a Cadiere in arm 1 retracting the stomach and the bedside assistant providing countertraction. A fenestrated bipolar is used in arm 2, and the vessel sealer is used in arm 4 (**Fig. 8**). During division of the

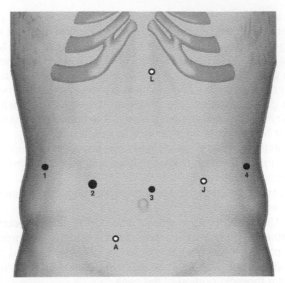

Fig. 7. Robotic port placement for abdominal dissection and conduit creation, with numbered robotic ports, and assistant (A), liver retractor (L), and J tube sites (J) indicated. (*Adapted from* BodyParts3D, licensed under CC Attribution-Share Alike 2.1 Japan. Available at: https://creativecommons.org/licenses/by-sa/2.1/jp/deed.en_US.)

gastropancreatic folds and transverse mesocolon dissection, hook cautery or monopolar scissors can also be used in arm 4 for dissection (**Fig. 9**).

Duodenal mobilization is performed with the vessel sealer with a combination of blunt dissection and sealing function.

The right gastric dissection is performed using arms 1 and 2 for retraction and the vessel sealer for dissection and division of the vessel (**Fig. 10**).

The left gastric dissection is performed with a combination of the hook and vessel sealer in arm 4. Traction is provided by grasping the left gastric pedicle with arm 1 and retracting toward the abdominal wall, while the assistant places a grasper posterior to the stomach to lift it toward the abdominal wall and slightly inferiorly (**Fig. 11**).

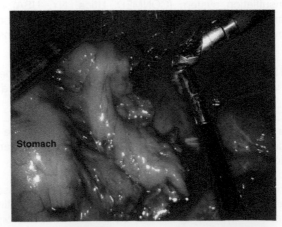

Fig. 8. Robotic greater curve dissection.

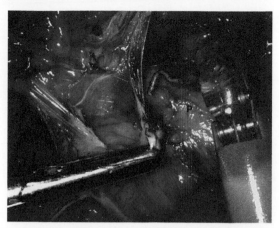

Fig. 9. Robotic dissection of the gastropancreatic folds separating stomach from pancreas (P).

The left gastric vein can be clipped by the assistant or divided with the vessel sealer. The left gastric artery is divided using the robotic stapler in arm 2.

The gastric conduit is created using multiple fires of the robotic stapler with 60-mm green loads in arm 2 (**Fig. 12**). The authors typically change the atraumatic grasper to arm 4 because it is used to manipulate the conduit, and fenestrated bipolar in arm 1 on the specimen. If there is difficulty using the robotic stapler due to thick tissue, a smaller bite can be taken to start the staple line. Alternatively, the assistant port can be upsized to accommodate the Endo GIA.

For TH-MIE, dissection into the mediastinum is performed using arm 1 to retract tissue anterior to the esophagus. The assistant provides traction by pulling the stomach down into the abdomen. Arm 2 is used to retract the esophagus side to side, or anteriorly and posteriorly, while a vessel sealer in arm 4 is used for blunt dissection and sealing. Alternatively, downward traction on the specimen can be provided by arm 1 while the assistant provides traction closer to the area of dissection (**Fig. 13**). As dissection proceeds superiorly, a 0° scope is used to aid in visualization. Posterior vascular and lymphatic branches are clipped by the assistant before division with the vessel sealer.

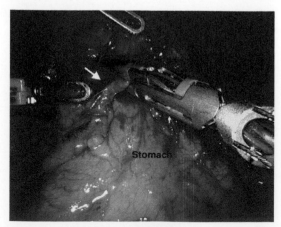

Fig. 10. Robotic right gastric artery (*arrow*) dissection.

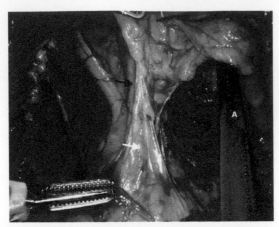

Fig. 11. Robotic celiac axis and left gastric pedicle lymphadenectomy. Retraction is provided by the assistant grasper (A), and the left gastric vein (*white arrow*) and left gastric pedicle (*black arrow*) are indicated.

The robotic platform has fluorescence imaging capability with Firefly, so the authors routinely perform intraoperative fluorescence imaging to evaluate the conduit during robotic cases (**Fig. 14**). Indocyanine green is reconstituted with 25 mg in 10 mL sterile water, and 3 mL of the solution is injected intravenously, followed by a saline flush. Note is made if the tip of the conduit appears poorly perfused, because this area can be excised after performing the anastomosis.

For patients requiring a jejunostomy tube placement, the robot is redocked to facilitate this portion of the operation (**Fig. 15**). The subxiphoid liver retractor site and assistant port are replaced with 8-mm robotic ports. Arm 1 is docked to the liver retractor site; arm 2 is docked to the right lateral port (previously arm 1), and arm 3 is docked at the previous assistant port site. Arm 4 is not used, and the prior 12-mm robotic port is used by the assistant. The jejunal enterotomy is created with a hook in arm 3, and the T-tube is inserted. A purse-string stitch is placed using the robotic needle drivers. After the tube is passed through the abdominal wall, the lateral transfascial stitch is placed and passed with the Carter-Thomason device (Cooper Surgical, Trumbull, CT, USA) to

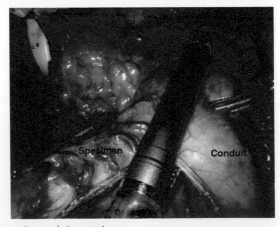

Fig. 12. Robotic gastric conduit creation.

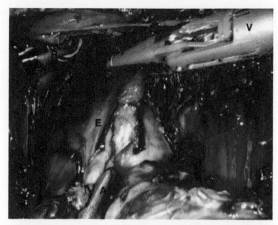

Fig. 13. Robotic transhiatal mediastinal dissection. Retraction is provided by the assistant (A) and robotic arm (R), whereas the robotic vessel sealer (V) is used to dissect the esophagus (E).

secure the bowel to the abdominal wall. The remaining stitches superiorly, medially, inferiorly, proximally, and distally are placed using the robotic needle drivers, securing seromuscular bites of the bowel to the abdominal wall (**Fig. 16**). The insufflation pressure can be lowered to facilitate apposition of the jejunum to the abdominal wall. Alternatively, if the mesentery is heavy or short, a distal transfascial suture can be placed to help hold the bowel anteriorly while the sutures are placed around the tube.

Thoracic Operation: Thoracoscopic

Positioning
The patient is positioned in a left lateral decubitus position with the bed flexed. The anterior superior iliac spine should be just below the break of the bed before flexing. A beanbag is placed under the patient for positioning, and an axillary roll is used. All pressure points should be padded. Both arms are flexed at 90° to 120°.

Ports
The optical entry camera port is inserted just below the tip of the scapula in the mid-axillary line; the surgeon's right hand is a 12-mm port placed just above the diaphragm

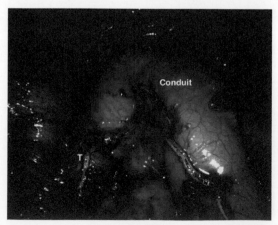

Fig. 14. Robotic fluorescence imaging using Firefly to evaluate perfusion of the conduit and the tip (T).

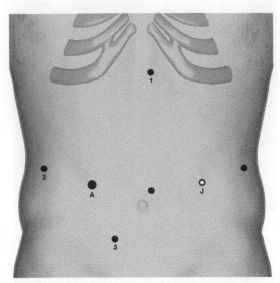

Fig. 15. Port placement for robotic jejunostomy tube placement, which requires redocking of the robot for use of arms 1 to 3 and an assistant (A) as indicated. (*Adapted from* BodyParts3D, licensed under CC Attribution-Share Alike 2.1 Japan. Available at: https:// creativecommons.org/licenses/by-sa/2.1/jp/deed.en_US.)

in line with the camera port, and the surgeon's left hand is midway between these 2 ports and slightly posterior (**Fig. 17**). A 12-mm assistant port is placed one rib above and anterior to the camera port. For IL-MIE, an additional anterior 5-mm assistant port is placed 3 rib spaces below the 12-mm assistant port.

Instruments
Instruments included Enseal, atraumatic graspers, Maryland dissector, gastric band dissector, Endo GIA, 5-mm 0° and 30° laparoscope, fan retractor, and 5-mm clip applier.

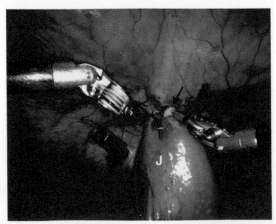

Fig. 16. Robotic jejunostomy tube placement, showing placement of the medial stitch securing the jejunum (J) to the abdominal wall, with J-tube (*arrow*) visible.

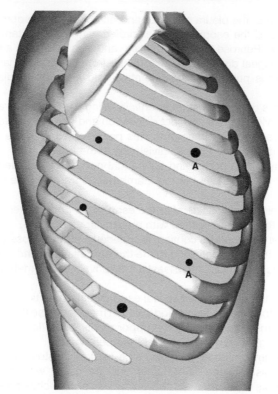

Fig. 17. Thoracoscopic port placement with 2 assistant ports (A) for IL-MIE. For a McKeown approach, only the superior assistant port is placed. (*Adapted from* BodyParts3D, licensed under CC Attribution-Share Alike 2.1 Japan. Available at: https://creativecommons.org/licenses/by-sa/2.1/jp/deed.en_US.)

Operation

The thoracic portion of the case is performed first for a McKeown MIE and is performed after the abdominal portion for IL-MIE. Representative intraoperative images of critical portions of the operation are included in the subsequent section describing the robotic approach.

Both the camera operator and the surgeon stand on the patient's right side (posterior), and an assistant stands on the patient's left side. The assistant controls one port for McKeown MIE and 2 ports for IL-MIE.

The position of the endotracheal tube is verified by bronchoscopy and the right lung is collapsed.

Access is obtained using optical entry technique with a 5-mm port just below the tip of the scapula. Additional ports are placed under direct vision. The thorax is insufflated with CO_2 to 8 mm Hg.

A fan retractor is introduced through the superior assistant port to retract the lung and help expose the esophagus. This retractor is adjusted throughout dissection for appropriate traction and exposure. In most patients, a 12-mm fan is needed. However, in some thin patients without lung disease, a 5-mm port and smaller fan suffice.

The esophageal dissection starts inferiorly and proceeds superiorly. The inferior pulmonary ligament is divided up to the pulmonary vein.

For McKeown MIE, the pleura posterior and anterior to the esophagus are divided with the Enseal, and the esophagus is encircled with the assistance of the gastric band dissector. A Penrose drain is passed and secured with an Endoloop. For IL-MIE, the esophageal dissection can continue from the abdominal dissection, and the Penrose drain is pulled into the operative field after the mediastinal pleural is divided.

The esophagus is dissected circumferentially using the Penrose drain for retraction, and the Enseal device is used for blunt dissection and to divide attachments circumferentially. Vascular and lymphatic branches posteriorly and to the right side of the esophagus should be clipped before division with the Enseal.

Paraesophageal lymph nodes and subcarinal nodes are included with the specimen, taking care to avoid injury to the membranous trachea. The vagus nerves are divided.

The azygous vein traverses lateral to the esophagus from posterior to anterior and should be dissected out and divided with a vascular staple load.

The esophageal dissection is continued superiorly, staying close to the esophagus to avoid injury to the RLN, continuing to the thoracic inlet and underneath the subclavian vessels for McKeown MIE and a least 5 cm above the proximal extent of the tumor for IL-MIE.

For McKeown MIE, most of the cervical esophageal dissection is completed under direct vision from the thoracoscopic ports, which may decrease the chance of injury to the RLN. The Penrose drain is left in the upper mediastinum/lower cervical region for later retrieval during the cervical phase of the operation.

For IL-MIE, the authors prefer a stapled side-to-side anastomosis and reserve end-to-side anastomosis with the EEA stapler only for cases with inadequate conduit length.[26] The authors experience has shown low leak and stricture rates using a stapled side-to-side anastomosis.[14] The esophagus is transected with a 60-mm Endo GIA with 3.5-mm staple height after the NGT is pulled back by the anesthesia team. The specimen with attached gastric conduit is pulled into the chest. The securing sutures are cut, and the specimen is extracted by enlarging the anterior assistant port and placing an Alexis wound protector (Applied Medical, Rancho Santa Margarita, CA, USA). Typically, a 3-cm incision is required on the skin, and the intercostal space is opened for 2 to 3 finger-breaths. The esophageal margin is examined by frozen section to ensure it is cancer free before performing the esophagogastrostomy. The cap for the Alexis is placed, which enables use of the 12-mm assistant port. The conduit and attached omentum are pulled to the apex of the chest, maintaining the staple line in the anterior orientation. The anastomosis is created between the posterior aspect of the gastric conduit and anterior aspect of the esophagus. The NGT is advanced and directed toward the anterior aspect of the esophagus. An esophagotomy is made by cutting off a corner of the staple line, and the NGT is pulled into the field. A full-thickness 2-0 silk stitch is placed at the esophagotomy site to secure the mucosa to the muscular wall of the esophagus and is used for traction during the creation of the anastomosis. A gastrotomy is made 6 cm from the tip and on the posterior aspect of the conduit. A 60-mm Endo GIA load with 3.5-mm staple height is inserted with the staple cartridge in the conduit and anvil in the esophagus and fired from the surgeon's right hand. Care must be taken to avoid catching the NGT in the staple line. Following staple firing, the NGT is advanced through the anastomosis into the distal stomach and left just above the diaphragm. Three or 4 silk stitches are used to approximate the edges of the esophagotomy and gastrotomy and thereby close the common channel and serve as handles to allow for stapled excision of the gastric and esophageal entry sites. Multiple 45-mm staple loads with 4.8-mm staple height are fired from the assistant port to excise the common channel and the entire end of the stapled esophagus. Alternatively, the common channel can be closed with meticulously placed and interrupted 2-0 Vicryl endostitches. Reinforcing U-stitches are placed at the crossing staple lines and a simple stitch is placed at the apex of the anastomosis to decrease tension on the staple line. The tip of the gastric conduit is excised with a stapler. The stomach is then secured at its posterior-superior aspect to the cut edge of the pleura with a silk stitch. An esophagogastroduodenoscopy (EGD) is performed to examine the anastomosis and perform a leak test. The omentum is secured over the anastomosis. The NGT position should be verified to be in the gastric conduit. The conduit is pushed back down through the hiatus to reduce any redundant conduit. It is then sutured to the left crus.

If it is anticipated that an EEA anastomosis will be performed, the specimen is extracted by upsizing the surgeon's left hand port so that the EEA stapler can be placed at this location in line with the esophagus and the gastric conduit. The anvil is secured in the cut end of the esophagus with the assistance of the Endo Stitch.

Intercostal nerve blocks are performed using long-acting or liposomal bupivacaine, and epidural catheters are rarely used. A 24-French Blake drain is left posteriorly and connected to suction at −20 cm H_2O; the lung is reinflated, and the incisions are closed.

Thoracic Operation: Robotic

Positioning
The patient is positioned with the left lateral decubitus with either a beanbag or a Pink Pad, bed flexed, and axillary roll in place.

Ports
Ports included three 8-mm and one 12-mm robotic ports, and one 12-mm assistant port (**Fig. 18**).

Instruments
Instruments included Cadiere, fenestrated bipolar, vessel sealer, needle drivers, Endo GIA, stapler, 30° scope, and 5-mm endoclips.

Operation

The operation proceeds in similar fashion to the thoracoscopic approach, and this section highlights only the deviations and considerations for the robotic approach.

A 30° scope is used via arm 3. Division of the inferior pulmonary ligament and dissection of the esophagus are carried out with retraction provided by arm 1 posteriorly and the assistant anteriorly. Dissection is performed using a fenestrated bipolar in arm 2 and vessel sealer or hook in arm 4. The esophagus is mobilized with assistance of the Penrose drain for traction (**Fig. 19**), and posterior lymphatics are clipped before division (**Fig. 20**).

The azygous vein can be dissected with the Maryland dissector in arm 4 and stapled with the robotic stapler via arm 2 (**Fig. 21**).

Division of the esophagus is performed by the assistant with an Endo GIA.

The specimen is extracted by enlarging the assistant port.

A stapled side-to-side anastomosis is routinely used and can be performed thoracoscopically by undocking arms 1 and 2, in identical fashion to the laparoscopic technique described in the previous section. The anastomosis is created with a 60-mm Endo GIA load with 3.5-mm staple height (**Fig. 22**), and the common gastrotomy and esophagotomy and stapled end of the esophagus are excised by the assistant with Endo GIA staple loads with 4.5-mm staple height (**Fig. 23**). Alternatively, the anastomosis can be created robotically using a 60-mm blue load, and the

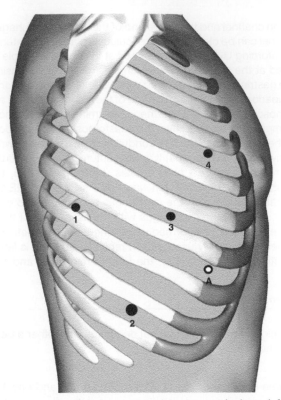

Fig. 18. Robotic thoracic port placement. A, assistant port. (*Adapted from* BodyParts3D, licensed under CC Attribution-Share Alike 2.1 Japan. Available at: https://creativecommons. org/licenses/by-sa/2.1/jp/deed.en_US.)

common channel is closed using 2-0 V-Loc absorbable sutures (Medtronic) (**Fig. 24**). Reinforcing stitches are typically placed in the thoracoscopic approach using the robotic needle drivers, with the sutures passed in via the assistant port or 12-mm robotic port.

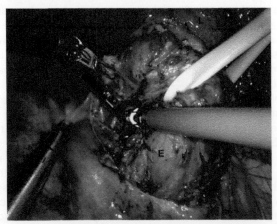

Fig. 19. Robotic esophageal mobilization with anterior traction on the Penrose drain. The esophagus (E) and lung (L) are visible.

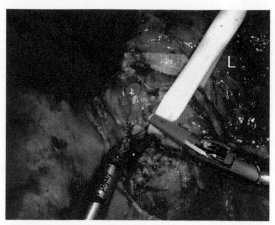

Fig. 20. Posterior lymphatics are clipped before division. L, lung.

Cervical Dissection

Positioning
The patient is positioned supine, neck extended, with a shoulder roll in place, and head turned slightly to the right.

Operation
An oblique incision is made overlying the anterior border of the left sternocleidomastoid muscle (SCM), extending to the sternal notch. The platysma is divided.

The SCM is dissected free and retracted laterally. The inferior belly of the omohyoid is divided. The internal jugular vein and carotid artery are retracted laterally. Crossing branches of the jugular vein are ligated.

The RLN is identified in the tracheoesophageal groove and kept up with the trachea. The prevertebral fascia is opened, and the esophagus is circumferentially isolated using blunt dissection.

For McKeown MIE, minimal dissection of the esophagus is necessary from the cervical approach. If adequate dissection is performed from the thoracic approach, the Penrose drain placed during the thoracic mobilization is easily pulled into the neck

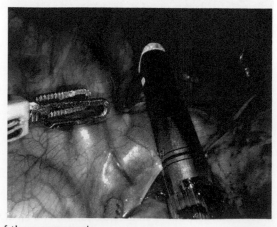

Fig. 21. Division of the azygous vein.

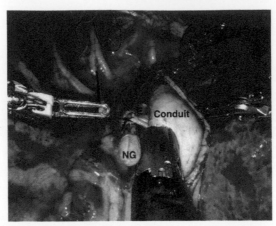

Fig. 22. Stapled side-to-side anastomosis between the esophagus (E) and conduit with the robotic stapler (S). NG, nasogastric tube.

incision, ensuring that the esophagus is free circumferentially. For a TH-MIE, the esophagus must be fully dissected and encircled from the cervical approach. Further dissection to accomplish complete esophageal mobilization from the abdomen to the neck must be carried into the mediastinum using a long blunt curved clamp, which is passed anterior and then posterior to the esophagus until the planes meet with the transhiatal dissection (**Fig. 25**). Remaining lateral attachments are divided from below.

Once the esophagus is completely mobilized, the specimen and gastric conduit are pulled out of the cervical incision before anastomosis.

A side-to-side stapled anastomosis is created after the NGT is pulled back by the anesthesia team. The conduit and esophagus are pulled out of the patient toward the surgeon so that the planned anastomosis is between the posterior conduit and anteromedial esophagus. The esophagus is not divided before anastomosis. An esophagotomy and gastrostomy are created, and the anastomosis is created with a fire of a 60-mm Endo GIA load with 3.5-mm staple height, with the anvil in the esophagus. The NGT is advanced and passed into the gastric conduit. The common

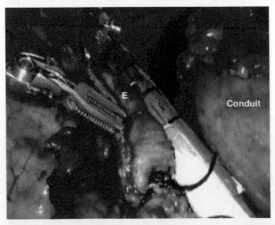

Fig. 23. Closure of the common gastrotomy and esophagotomy and tip of the esophagus (E) by stapled excision.

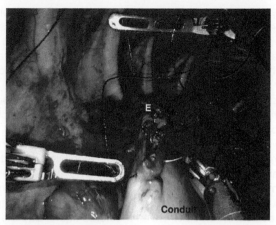

Fig. 24. Closure of common gastrotomy and esophagotomy with V-Loc sutures. E, esophagus.

enterotomy and the end of the gastric conduit and the entire esophagus are stapled using one fire of a 60-mm TA stapler with 3.5-mm staple height. The crotch of the anastomosis is reinforced with 2 interrupted seromuscular bites using the TA staple handle for retraction purposes. Following this, the esophagus and the apex of the gastric conduit are divided flush with the TA stapler, and specimens are sent to pathology. The TA staple line is imbricated with 3-0 PDS (polydioxanone; Ethicon) in a running fashion.

The anastomosis is returned to the mediastinum, and excess conduit is pulled down from the abdomen.

A 7-French Jackson-Pratt drain is placed into the superior mediastinum. The platysma and skin are closed.

POSTOPERATIVE MANAGEMENT

The authors used an enhanced recovery pathway derived from evidence-based practice.[27] Patients are typically admitted to a step-down unit with telemetry monitoring on

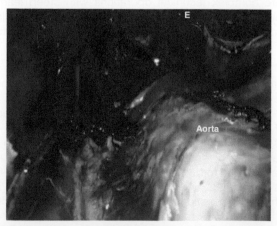

Fig. 25. Robotic transhiatal dissection posterior to the esophagus (E) meeting with a clamp from the cervical dissection.

postoperative day (POD) 0 and transferred to a regular nursing floor on POD 1. Patients routinely receive intravenous acetaminophen and narcotics via a patient-controlled analgesic pump. The authors sometimes use ketorolac but limit doses due to bleeding and nephrotoxicity risk. Patients are out of bed starting on POD 1 and ambulate with the assistance of a physical therapist initially, and eventually with an aide, nurse, or family member.

Chest radiographs (CXRs) are obtained daily to monitor for conduit distension and pulmonary complications.[28] Early conduit dilation suggests malfunction of the NGT, which is flushed or repositioned accordingly.

Tube feeds are started on POD 2 and advanced to goal with return of bowel function. The NGT is removed on POD 3 if CXR shows a collapsed conduit.

Patients with an intrathoracic anastomosis undergo either an esophagram with water-soluble contrast or a CT esophagram on POD 4. Diet is advanced to clear liquids if there is no leak or obstruction. Patients with a cervical anastomosis undergo bedside swallow evaluation on POD 4 with a colored liquid, and diet is advanced to clear liquids if there is no evidence of aspiration or leakage via the neck drain. For patients with a hoarse voice or concern for aspiration, a formal evaluation by speech language pathology is performed. Diet is advanced to full liquids the day after clear liquids. The neck drain is removed POD 4 if there is no evidence of a leak.

Chest tubes are removed on POD 5 if no air or chyle leak.

Patients are discharged on POD 6 to 7 on a full liquid diet to meet 50% of nutritional needs and nocturnal tube feeds to meet the remaining requirements. All patients are evaluated by a registered dietician preoperatively, during hospitalization, and at postoperative visits.

Patients are seen in clinic 1 to 2 weeks after discharge with a CXR as clinically indicated. If the conduit appears within expected limits and the patient is tolerating full liquids, then the diet is liberalized to soft foods, and the patient is instructed to decrease and ultimately stop tube feeds. Patients are seen every 2 to 3 weeks, and if they are tolerating an oral diet without significant weight loss, then the jejunostomy tube is removed.

SUMMARY

Esophageal and GEJ cancers can represent difficult oncologic and surgical problems. MIE or RAMIE are complex technical operations with steep learning curves but currently are the surgical treatment of choice for these tumors. Establishment of a systematic intraoperative and postoperative approach can optimize outcomes.

REFERENCES

1. Siegel RL, Miller KD, Jemal A. Cancer statistics, 2018. CA Cancer J Clin 2018; 68(1):7–30.
2. Malhotra GK, Yanala U, Ravipati A, et al. Global trends in esophageal cancer. J Surg Oncol 2017;115(5):564–79.
3. de Oliveira C, Bremner KE, Pataky R, et al. Understanding the costs of cancer care before and after diagnosis for the 21 most common cancers in Ontario: a population-based descriptive study. CMAJ Open 2013;1(1):E1–8.
4. van Hagen P, Hulshof MC, van Lanschot JJ, et al. Preoperative chemoradiotherapy for esophageal or junctional cancer. N Engl J Med 2012;366(22):2074–84.
5. Cunningham D, Allum WH, Stenning SP, et al. Perioperative chemotherapy versus surgery alone for resectable gastroesophageal cancer. N Engl J Med 2006; 355(1):11–20.

6. Al-Batran S, Homann N, Schmalenberg H, et al. Perioperative chemotherapy with docetaxel, oxaliplatin, and fluorouracil/leucovorin (FLOT) versus epirubicin, cisplatin, and fluorouracil or capecitabine (ECF/ECX) for resectable gastric or gastroesophageal junction (GEJ) adenocarcinoma (FLOT4-AIO): a multicenter, randomized phase 3 trial. J Clin Oncol 2017;35(Suppl 15):S4004.

7. Kukar M, Hochwald SN. Special operative and multimodal therapy considerations in EGJ cancer care: western viewpoints. In: Morita SY, Balch CM, Klimberg VS, et al, editors. Textbook of complex general surgical oncology. 1st edition. New York: McGraw-Hill Education; 2018. p. 985–94. Chapter 94.

8. Espinoza-Mercado F, Imai TA, Borgella JD, et al. Does the approach matter? Comparing survival in robotic, minimally invasive and open esophagectomies. Ann Thorac Surg 2018. https://doi.org/10.1016/j.athoracsur.2018.08.039.

9. Biere SS, van Berge Henegouwen MI, Maas KW, et al. Minimally invasive versus open oesophagectomy for patients with oesophageal cancer: a multicentre, open-label, randomised controlled trial. Lancet 2012;379(9829):1887–92.

10. Straatman J, van der Wielen N, Cuesta MA, et al. Minimally invasive versus open esophageal resection: three-year follow-up of the previously reported randomized controlled trial: the TIME trial. Ann Surg 2017;266(2):232–6.

11. van der Sluis PC, van der Horst S, May AM, et al. Robot-assisted minimally invasive thoraco-laparoscopic esophagectomy versus open transthoracic esophagectomy for resectable esophageal cancer: a randomized controlled trial. J Clin Oncol 2018;36(suppl 4S) [abstract: 6].

12. Luketich JD, Pennathur A, Awais O, et al. Outcomes after minimally invasive esophagectomy: review of over 1000 patients. Ann Surg 2012;256(1):95–103.

13. Kassis ES, Kosinski AS, Ross P, et al. Predictors of anastomotic leak after esophagectomy: an analysis of the society of thoracic surgeons general thoracic database. Ann Thorac Surg 2013;96(6):1919–26.

14. Ben-David K, Tuttle R, Kukar M, et al. Minimally invasive esophagectomy utilizing a stapled side-to-side anastomosis is safe in the western patient population. Ann Surg Oncol 2016;23(9):3056–62.

15. van der Sluis PC, Ruurda JP, Verhage RJ, et al. Oncologic long-term results of robot-assisted minimally invasive thoraco-laparoscopic esophagectomy with two-field lymphadenectomy for esophageal cancer. Ann Surg Oncol 2015; 22(Suppl 3):S1350–6.

16. van Workum F, van der Maas J, van den Wildenberg FJ, et al. Improved functional results after minimally invasive esophagectomy: intrathoracic versus cervical anastomosis. Ann Thorac Surg 2017;103(1):267–73.

17. van Workum F, Bouwense SA, Luyer MD, et al. Intrathoracic versus Cervical ANastomosis after minimally invasive esophagectomy for esophageal cancer: study protocol of the ICAN randomized controlled trial. Trials 2016;17(1):505.

18. Montenovo MI, Chambers K, Pellegrini CA, et al. Outcomes of laparoscopic-assisted transhiatal esophagectomy for adenocarcinoma of the esophagus and esophago-gastric junction. Dis Esophagus 2011;24(6):430–6.

19. Dunn DH, Johnson EM, Morphew JA, et al. Robot-assisted transhiatal esophagectomy: a 3-year single-center experience. Dis Esophagus 2013;26(2):159–66.

20. Parry K, Ruurda JP, van der Sluis PC, et al. Current status of laparoscopic transhiatal esophagectomy for esophageal cancer patients: a systematic review of the literature. Dis Esophagus 2017;30(1):1–7.

21. van Workum F, Stenstra MHBC, Berkelmans GHK, et al. Learning curve and associated morbidity of minimally invasive esophagectomy: a retrospective multicenter study. Ann Surg 2017. https://doi.org/10.1097/SLA.0000000000002469.

22. Park S, Hyun K, Lee HJ, et al. A study of the learning curve for robotic oesopha-gectomy for oesophageal cancer. Eur J Cardiothorac Surg 2018;53(4):862–70.

23. Zhang H, Chen L, Wang Z, et al. The Learning Curve for Robotic McKeown Esophagectomy in patients with esophageal cancer. Ann Thorac Surg 2018; 105(4):1024–30.

24. Hochwald SN, Ben-David K. Minimally invasive esophagectomy with cervical esophagogastric anastomosis. J Gastrointest Surg 2012;16(9):1775–81.

25. Ben-David K, Kim T, Caban AM, et al. Pre-therapy laparoscopic feeding jejunos-tomy is safe and effective in patients undergoing minimally invasive esophagec-tomy for cancer. J Gastrointest Surg 2013;17(8):1352–8.

26. Ben-David K, Sarosi GA, Cendan JC, et al. Technique of minimally invasive Ivor Lewis esophagogastrectomy with intrathoracic stapled side-to-side anastomosis. J Gastrointest Surg 2010;14(10):1613–8.

27. Low DE, Allum W, De Manzoni G, et al. Guidelines for perioperative care in esophagectomy: enhanced recovery after surgery (ERAS). World J Surg 2018. https://doi.org/10.1007/s00268-018-4786-4.

28. Gabriel E, Shah R, Attwood K, et al. The first postesophagectomy chest X-ray predicts respiratory failure and the need for tracheostomy. J Surg Res 2018; 224:89–96.

Minimally Invasive Gastric Cancer Surgery

Christina L. Costantino, MD[a], John T. Mullen, MD[b],*

KEYWORDS

- Gastric cancer • Minimally invasive surgery • Laparoscopic gastrectomy
- Robotic gastrectomy

KEY POINTS

- Short-term outcomes demonstrate that laparoscopic gastrectomy is safe in the hands of experienced surgeons; however, longer term outcomes are necessary to definitively determine its oncologic equivalency to traditional open gastrectomy.
- Minimally invasive techniques, including laparoscopic and robotic surgery, have a minimum learning curve required to achieve proficiency.
- Patients well-selected for minimally invasive gastrectomy may experience decreased morbidity compared with open surgery.

INTRODUCTION

Gastric cancer represents the third leading cause of cancer-related deaths worldwide, with the highest reported mortality rates in eastern Asia and the lowest in North America.[1] There is also wide variation in the incidence of gastric cancer worldwide, with more than 70% of new gastric cancers diagnosed in developing countries.[1] Although the incidence of new gastric cancer cases overall in the United States has decreased by about 1.5% per year in each of the last 10 years,[2] there has been a 70% increase in the incidence of noncardia, distal gastric cancers in the 25- to 39-year-old population in the United States over the past few years.[3]

The majority of data concerning the surgical management of gastric cancer published in the past several decades has been generated from East Asia. Guidelines for the optimal management of surgically resectable disease are based on their experience,[4] including detailed definitions of the regional nodal basins and the optimal extent of lymphadenectomy, as well as short- and long-term outcomes from

Disclosure statement: No financial disclosures.

[a] Department of Surgery, Massachusetts General Hospital, GRB-425, 55 Fruit Street, Boston, MA 02114, USA; [b] Department of Surgery, Massachusetts General Hospital, Yawkey Center for Outpatient Care, 32 Fruit Street, YAW-7-7926, Boston, MA 02114, USA
* Corresponding author.
E-mail address: JMULLEN@mgh.harvard.edu

treatments ranging from the endoscopic resection of early gastric cancers to the radical resection with D2 lymphadenectomy of advanced gastric cancers. Given the increased incidence and heightened awareness of gastric cancer in countries like Japan and Korea, endoscopic screening has led to earlier diagnosis, with approximately 50% of patients diagnosed with early gastric cancers.[5] This shift to the diagnosis of gastric cancer at a much earlier stage, together with dramatic advances in surgical technology, have permitted Asian surgeons to introduce and refine less invasive surgical approaches to the treatment of gastric cancer.

In the past decade, there has been increasing effort to generate level I evidence to support the notion that minimally invasive gastrectomy is oncologically equivalent to open gastrectomy, while offering patients a less morbid, faster recovery from surgery. This growing body of data from both the East and West suggests that minimally invasive surgery may be the preferred option for the surgical treatment of gastric cancer in well-selected patient populations. This article reviews the evidence comparing laparoscopic with open gastrectomy for early and advanced gastric cancers, the current status of robotic gastrectomy, and the learning curves associated with minimally invasive gastrectomy.

LAPAROSCOPIC GASTRECTOMY FOR EARLY GASTRIC CANCER

Kitano and colleagues[6] performed the first laparoscopic-assisted gastrectomy for gastric cancer in 1994, and since then there has been the widespread adoption of minimally invasive techniques for the treatment of gastric cancer worldwide. This has been particularly true in the countries of Japan and Korea, where now more than one-half of all gastrectomies are performed laparoscopically. The more rapid adoption of minimally invasive surgery for gastric cancer in Japan and Korea is in large part owing to the high incidence rates of gastric cancer overall, and of early stage gastric cancer, in these countries.

Regardless of the technical approach, the goals of surgery for gastric cancer include the following: achieving a complete (R0) resection with negative microscopic margins, performing an adequate lymph node dissection, minimizing the risk (morbidity) to the patient, and optimizing long-term quality of life.[5] The ultimate metrics for the adoption of minimally invasive techniques in place of traditional open surgery for the treatment of any cancer is the demonstration of equivalency (if not superiority) in both safety and oncologic efficacy and, in the case of gastric cancer, there is a rapidly growing body of evidence in support of minimally invasive techniques.[7]

The first randomized, controlled trial comparing laparoscopic distal gastrectomy with traditional open distal gastrectomy (ODG) was a small study of 28 patients published in 2002 by Kitano and colleagues[8] All patients had early gastric cancer and underwent Billroth I reconstruction. These investigators reported that patients undergoing laparoscopic-assisted distal gastrectomy (LADG) compared with open gastrectomy (**Table 1**) experienced less intraoperative blood loss, less postoperative pain, earlier recovery, and, importantly, an equivalent oncologic operation.[8] Over the past decade, several large, nonrandomized studies, primarily from centers of excellence in East Asia, have reported similar outcomes for minimally invasive gastrectomy compared with open gastrectomy.[9–13]

The majority of surgeons in the East now use laparoscopic gastrectomy for clinical T1N0 disease that is not endoscopically resectable.[5] More recent prospective, randomized trials have generated level 1 evidence that minimally invasive gastrectomy is at least equivalent, if not superior, to open gastrectomy in outcomes such as length of stay, postoperative pain, and intraoperative blood loss. However, these trials have

Table 1
Selected nonrandomized clinical trials comparing laparoscopic, robotic, and open gastrectomy for gastric cancer

Author, Year	Procedure Type and Number of Patients	Total Number of Patients	Decreased Operative Time	Greater Number of LNs Retrieved	Decreased EBL	Decreased LOS	Decreased Overall Morbidity Rate	Mortality Rate
Kim et al,[55] 2005	LADG 71 ODG 147	219	ODG	Equivalent	—	LADG	Equivalent	Equivalent
Hur et al,[32] 2008	LADG 26 ODG 25	51	ODG	—	LADG	Equivalent	Equivalent	—
Yoo et al,[19] 2009	LADG 102 ODG 71	173	ODG	ODG	Equivalent	LADG	Equivalent	Equivalent
Strong et al,[21] 2009	LG 30 OG 30	60	OG	Equivalent	Equivalent	LG	LG	—
Lee et al,[56] 2009	LADG 294 ODG 664	958	ODG	LADG	—	LADG	LADG	Equivalent
Du et al,[31] 2009	LADG 78 ODG 90	168	Equivalent	Equivalent	LADG	LADG	Equivalent	Equivalent
Hwang et al,[12] 2009	LADG 45 ODG 83	128	ODG	Equivalent	LADG	Equivalent	Equivalent	Equivalent
Guzman et al,[22] 2009	LG 22 OG 29	51	OG	Equivalent	LG	LG	Equivalent	Equivalent
Kunisaki et al,[11] 2009	LADG 130 ODG 81	211	ODG	Equivalent	LADG	LADG	Equivalent	Equivalent
Kim et al,[10] 2012	OG 4542 LG 861 RG 436	5839	OG	Equivalent	RG, LG	RG, LG	Equivalent	Equivalent
Suda et al,[57] 2015	LG 438 RG 88	526	LG	Equivalent	LG	RG	RG	Equivalent
Huang et al,[52] 2014	RG 72 LG 73	145	LG	Equivalent	Equivalent	Equivalent	Equivalent	Equivalent
Kelly et al,[20] 2015	LG 87 OG 87	174	OG	Equivalent	LG	LG	Equivalent	Equivalent
Kinoshita et al,[13] 2018	LG 305 OG 305	610	OG	LG	LG	LG	Equivalent	Equivalent

Abbreviations: EBL, estimated blood loss; LADG, laparoscopic-assisted distal gastrectomy; LG, laparoscopic gastrectomy; LN, lymph nodes; LOS, length of stay; ODG, open distal gastrectomy; OG, open gastrectomy; RG, robotic gastrectomy.

similarly consistently showed that minimally invasive gastrectomy is associated with an increase in operative time compared with open gastrectomy.[14–17]

In 2016, the Korean Laparoscopic Study Group (KLASS) published their findings of a multicenter, randomized, controlled trial to study differences in perioperative morbidity and mortality and overall survival in patients undergoing LADG versus those undergoing ODG for early gastric cancer.[15] Of the 1426 patients enrolled in this trial, 705 were assigned to the LADG group, and the analysis demonstrated that the overall complication rate was significantly lower in the LADG group (13.0%) than in the ODG group (19.9%; $P = .001$), primarily owing to a lower incidence of wound complications in the LADG group. The rates of major intraabdominal complications (7.6% vs 10.3%) and of mortality (0.6% vs 0.3%) were similar between the 2 groups. Importantly, however, the number of lymph nodes retrieved in the LADG group was significantly less than that of the ODG group (40.5 vs 43.7; $P>.001$).[15] Although both nodal yields were more than adequate for accurate pathologic staging, nodal yield is an important measure of oncologic equivalency and is an important consideration when adopting new surgical techniques for the treatment of gastric cancer.

Western countries have been slower to adopt a minimally invasive approach, likely owing to the lower incidence of gastric cancer overall, and of early gastric cancer in particular, in the West compared with the East. Laparoscopic gastrectomy is a technically demanding procedure, with a learning curve estimated to be somewhere in the range of 60 to 90 cases,[18,19] which for the average Western surgeon specializing in gastric cancer may take as long as 3 to 5 years to accrue. However, with a growing body of evidence demonstrating the feasibility and oncologic equivalency of minimally invasive gastrectomy to open gastrectomy, as well as the potential benefits of lower morbidity and a faster recovery, the technique is gaining increased popularity in the West.

Several nonrandomized reviews from Western centers over the past few decades have examined outcomes in patients undergoing laparoscopic versus open gastrectomy and have found that, for well-selected patients, laparoscopic gastrectomy is a safe and effective approach.[20–22] Specifically, Kelly and colleagues[20] found in a recent nonrandomized study that although laparoscopic procedures were associated with increased operative time, patients experienced decreased rates of early (27% vs 16%) and late (17% vs 7%) complications ($P<.01$), as well as less blood loss (100 mL vs 150 mL; $P<.01$). Importantly, patients undergoing laparoscopic procedures were more likely to receive adjuvant therapy (82% vs 51%; $P<.01$).[20]

In 2005, Huscher and colleagues[23] published the only prospective randomized trial to date in the West comparing 5-year clinical outcomes between laparoscopic and open surgery for gastric cancer. Operative mortality and morbidity rates were not significantly different between laparoscopic and open procedures. Further, there was no difference between groups in 5-year overall and disease-free survival rates. Additionally, patients experienced a shorter time to oral intake and a decreased length of stay.[23]

Several metaanalyses have summarized the available literature of randomized, controlled trials to date and have found that a minimally invasive approach to early gastric cancer is both safe and oncologically equivalent to an open procedure in well-selected patients and centers.[24–26] Moreover, minimally invasive techniques may also provide potential benefits, including a decrease in overall morbidity and blood loss.

LAPAROSCOPIC GASTRECTOMY FOR ADVANCED GASTRIC CANCER

Despite the growing literature to support the minimally invasive approach to early gastric cancer, the National Comprehensive Cancer Network and Japanese guidelines still indicate that the standard surgical treatment for advanced gastric cancer is an open gastrectomy with D2 lymphadenectomy.[4,27] The laparoscopic approach to advanced gastric cancer is technically more challenging given the complexities of the lymph node dissection and concerns about the completeness of resection of bulky, locally advanced tumors. Despite these added technical challenges, several centers in Asia have published nonrandomized studies demonstrating the safety and oncologic efficacy of minimally invasive gastrectomy for advanced gastric cancer.[12,28–30] Specifically, Hwang and colleagues[12] compared 47 patients undergoing LADG with 83 patients undergoing ODG and concluded that LADG with extended lymphadenectomy for advanced gastric cancer was feasible and safe, although it was associated with a longer operative time. However, the LADG cohort experienced significantly lower rates of morbidity and mortality in addition to a shorter postoperative recovery time. In terms of oncologic equivalence, there were no differences in the rates of proximal margin positivity or in the mean number of lymph nodes examined between the LADG and ODG groups.[12]

More recently, Kinoshita and colleagues[13] published a large multicenter review of patients who underwent either open gastrectomy (n = 305) or laparoscopic gastrectomy (n = 305) for locally advanced gastric cancer between 2008 and 2014. They reported no differences in the 5-year survival rates (53.0% vs 54.2%) or recurrence rates (30.8% vs 29.8%) between the 2 groups, and both groups had similar patterns of recurrence.[13]

Based on the encouraging findings of several nonrandomized studies demonstrating the safety and efficacy of laparoscopic gastrectomy for advanced gastric cancer in Asia,[12,13,29,31,32] the first randomized, controlled trial to include patients with advanced gastric cancer was published in 2011.[33] Cai and colleagues[33] enrolled 123 patients, 61 of whom were randomized to laparoscopic-assisted gastrectomy. The laparoscopic group had significantly longer operative times (267.9 ± 54.3 min in the LAG group vs 182.0 ± 41.0 min in the open gastrectomy group; $P<.0001$) but had less intraoperative blood loss. There was no significant difference in the overall postoperative morbidity rate (12.2% in the LAG group and 19.2% in the open gastrectomy group; $P = .357$), although pulmonary infections were observed more frequently in the open gastrectomy cohort. Importantly, they found no statistically significant difference in the overall survival rate between the laparoscopic and open groups.[33]

Hu and colleagues[34] recently published a randomized, controlled trial of patients undergoing laparoscopic distal gastrectomy with D2 lymphadenectomy (n = 519) compared with ODG with D2 lymphadenectomy (n = 520) in patients with advanced gastric cancer. They observed no significant differences in postoperative morbidity or mortality rates and concluded that in the hands of experienced surgeons, laparoscopic gastrectomy with D2 lymphadenectomy for advanced disease can be safely performed.

These data were supported by a recently published prospective, randomized controlled trial by Shi and colleagues[35] comparing short-term outcomes in 322 patients undergoing either laparoscopic (n = 162) or open (n = 160) gastrectomy with D2 lymphadenectomy for locally advanced gastric cancer. They reported a 3.7% conversion rate from the laparoscopic to the open approach. There was no difference in the overall complication rate between the laparoscopic and open groups (11.7% vs 14.4%, respectively; $P = .512$), and neither cohort experienced a perioperative death.[35] Given their experience, the authors concluded that these excellent short term outcomes justified the adoption of laparoscopic gastrectomy with extended lymphadenectomy for advanced gastric cancer at experienced centers (**Table 2**).

Table 2
Selected randomized, controlled clinical trials comparing LG and OG for gastric cancer

Author, Year	Procedure Type and Number of Patients	Total Number of Patients	Decreased Operative Time	Greater Number of LNs Retrieved	Decreased EBL	Decreased LOS	Decreased Overall Morbidity Rate	Mortality Rate
Kitano et al,[8] 2002	LADG 14 / ODG 14	28	ODG	Equivalent	LADG	Equivalent	Equivalent	Equivalent
Lee et al,[58] 2009	LADG 24 / ODG 23	47	ODG	Equivalent	Equivalent	Equivalent	LADG	—
Huscher et al,[23] 2005	LG 30 / OG 29	59	Equivalent	Equivalent	LG	LG	Equivalent	Equivalent
Hayashi et al,[59] 2005	LADG 14 / ODG 14	28	ODG	Equivalent	Equivalent	LADG	—	Equivalent
Kim et al,[53] 2008	LADG 82 / ODG 82	164	ODG	ODG	LADG	LADG	—	—
Kim et al,[60] 2010	LADG 179 / ODG 163	342	ODG	—	LADG	—	Equivalent	Equivalent
Cai et al,[33] 2011	LAG 61 / OG 62	123	OG	Equivalent	Equivalent	Equivalent	Equivalent	Equivalent
Takiguchi et al,[61] 2013	LADG 20 / ODG 20	40	ODG	Equivalent	LADG	LADG	—	—
Aoyama et al,[16] 2014	LADG 13 / ODG 13	26	ODG	Equivalent	LADG	—	Equivalent	Equivalent
Kim et al,[15] 2016	LADG 644 / ODG 612	1256	ODG	ODG	LADG	LADG	LADG	Equivalent
Hu et al,[34] 2016	LG 519 / OG 520	1039	OG	Equivalent	LG	LG	Equivalent	Equivalent
Shi et al,[35] 2018	LAG 162 / OG 160	322	ODG	Equivalent	LAG	LAG	Equivalent	Equivalent

Abbreviations: EBL, estimated blood loss; LADG, laparoscopic-assisted distal gastrectomy; LG, laparoscopic gastrectomy; LN, lymph nodes; LOS, length of stay; ODG, open distal gastrectomy; OG, open gastrectomy.

To gather more evidence in support of the minimally invasive approach to advanced gastric cancers, in 2012 the Korean Laparoscopic Gastrointestinal Surgery Study (KLASS-02) launched a multicenter, prospective, randomized, phase III trial to compare the efficacy of laparoscopic distal gastrectomy with D2 lymph node dissection with conventional open surgery. The primary study end point is the 3-year relapse-free survival rate, and secondary end points include the 3-year overall survival rate, postoperative morbidity and mortality rates, postoperative recovery index, and quality of life.[36] Additional multicenter trials evaluating the efficacy of laparoscopic gastrectomy for the treatment of gastric cancer are similarly ongoing in China and Japan (KLASS-03, JLSSG0901, CLASS-01) and in the West (STOMACH trial).[37]

Multiple metaanalyses of the collective literature to date comparing laparoscopic gastrectomy with open gastrectomy for advanced gastric cancer have been published, and all of them have concluded that the 2 techniques have similar outcomes, including similar lymph node yields and equivalent rates of recurrence and overall survival.[24,38–40] Vinuela and colleagues[24] published the most comprehensive and stringent metaanalysis to date, summarizing the outcomes of minimally invasive gastrectomy for both early and advanced gastric cancers. Between 2000 and 2009, 38 studies were identified that met their eligibility criteria, including 6 randomized and 19 nonrandomized controlled trials composed of a total of 3055 patients (n = 1658 laparoscopic distal gastrectomy and n = 1397 open distal gastrectomy). Although laparoscopic distal gastrectomy was associated with a longer operative time, it was associated with a lower overall complication rate, fewer medical complications, fewer minor surgical complications, less blood loss, and a shorter hospital stay. Although patients in the open distal gastrectomy group had a significantly greater mean number of lymph nodes harvested, the groups had similar percentages of patients who had at least 15 lymph nodes examined.[24] The long-term significance of these differences in lymph node yield between the minimally invasive and open surgical procedures is unclear given the paucity of long-term survival data.

The importance of the extent of lymph node dissection and the potential survival advantage that it confers for patients with gastric cancer has been extensively studied and debated.[41] The Japanese Gastric Cancer Association has defined the lymph node stations about the stomach and the regional vasculature as well as the indications for a D2 lymphadenectomy.[5] It is recommended that at least 16 lymph nodes be pathologically examined for optimal assignment of an accurate nodal (N) stage.[42] An adequate lymph node dissection has been deemed essential not only for accurate staging, but also for the prevention of locoregional recurrence and, though certainly open to debate, for optimal long-term survival.[5] Because the performance of a D1+ or a D2 lymph node dissection is perhaps the greatest challenge of the minimally invasive approach to gastric cancer, any study evaluating the efficacy of this procedure must include data about the nodal yield.

ROBOTIC GASTRECTOMY FOR GASTRIC CANCER

Since robotic surgery was first introduced into clinical practice in 2000, it has gained dramatic interest and rapid adoption in many fields of surgery. Experienced robotic surgeons have found the technology to be more technically versatile, especially for surgical cases of increased complexity.[43] Given its relatively nascent application to the surgical treatment of gastric cancer, there remains a dearth of trials evaluating its efficacy in both short- and long-term outcomes.

In 2003, Hashizume and Sugimachi[44] published the first report of robotic-assisted gastric surgery in patients with early stage gastric cancer. A few years later, Anderson and associates[45] published the first small series (n = 7) in the West of robotic-assisted laparoscopic subtotal gastrectomies with extended lymphadenectomy for early distal gastric cancers. Despite the small size of the series, they reported no operative mortality, an acceptable lymph node yield, and a median length of stay of just 4 days. Song and colleagues[46] published a larger report (n = 100) 2 years later comparing outcomes in robotic-assisted gastrectomy for early gastric cancer demonstrating its safety and feasibility in their cohort. They reported a 1% operative mortality rate and a 13% operative morbidity rate. Importantly, in all patients they were able to achieve an R0 resection and harvest a mean number of 36.7 lymph nodes.[46]

Pan and colleagues[47] performed a metaanalysis of 5 studies in the published literature evaluating the oncologic outcomes of robotic versus laparoscopic gastrectomy. Robotic gastrectomy was found to have equivalent oncologic outcomes to laparoscopic gastrectomy, including similar overall and disease-free survival rates and recurrence rates.

Chen and colleagues[48] recently published a metaanalysis to evaluate the safety, feasibility, and efficacy of robotic gastrectomy compared with laparoscopic gastrectomy. The authors included 5953 patients from a total of 19 studies, two of which were from Italy and the rest from East Asia. Robotic gastrectomy was associated with a longer operative time but with less blood loss and an earlier time to oral intake. There were no significant differences found with respect to length of hospital stay, morbidity or mortality rates, lymph node yields, or recurrence rates.[48] Owing to limited data, however, long-term survival rates could not be assessed. When performing subgroup analyses comparing the outcomes of robotic versus laparoscopic distal gastrectomy or robotic versus laparoscopic total gastrectomy, there were no significant differences between the groups. Importantly, the robotic technique was associated with a higher cost than the laparoscopic technique, primarily owing to the cost of the instrumentation and the longer operative time.

Ultimately, given the available published literature, robotic gastrectomy with extended lymphadenectomy can be considered a safe procedure with equivalent short-term oncologic outcomes (R0 resection rate and nodal yield) to either laparoscopic or open gastrectomy for the surgical treatment of gastric cancer.[49] More studies with longer term follow-up are needed to assess the equivalency of the robotic approach to other surgical approaches in terms of disease-free and overall survivals.

SURGEON EXPERIENCE AND PATIENT SELECTION FOR MINIMALLY INVASIVE GASTRECTOMY

Central to the evolution of surgical techniques and changes to the standard of care is the demonstration of equivalent, if not improved, patient outcomes. When applying the current evidence to the treatment of a given patient population, one must consider the inherent differences between Eastern and Western patients. For example, Western countries observe a higher percentage of advanced gastric cancer on presentation compared with Eastern countries, and this factor certainly contributes to the surgical complexity of a case and should inform the decision regarding the appropriateness of a minimally invasive approach for a given patient.[3] Additionally, Eastern patients tend to present with gastric cancer at a younger age than in the West, and they tend to have a lower body mass index and fewer medical comorbidities, all of which influence the decision making regarding the choice of surgical approach. Most surgeons would agree that the patients who are most suitable for a minimally invasive gastrectomy are those with a low body mass index, few comorbidities, and early stage cancers.

Additional factors that are essential to the preoperative evaluation and stratification of patients to the most appropriate surgical technique include endoscopic ultrasound and cross-sectional imaging with a high-quality, multiphasic computed tomography scan. Vascular anomalies, including an accessory or replaced left hepatic artery or a replaced common or right hepatic artery, should be examined through arterial phase imaging to assess the feasibility and safety of a minimally invasive approach.[5] Additionally, the planned method of gastrointestinal reconstruction (eg, Billroth I or II or Roux-en-Y) and whether it is to be done intracorporeally or extracorporeally is an important factor when considering a minimally invasive approach versus a conventional open approach.

One must also consider a patient's fitness for laparoscopic gastric surgery in terms of their medical comorbidities, including the ability to tolerate a pneumoperitoneum and a history of prior abdominal surgery.[5] Those patients with significant cardiopulmonary disease who might benefit from a shorter operative time may be best suited to the conventional open approach.[7] Moreover, these considerations must be weighed in the context of a given surgeon's experience level.[5] A strong consideration should be paid to the ability to achieve an adequate lymphadenectomy with a minimally invasive approach given the data in support of a potential survival benefit conferred by a more extensive lymphadenectomy, assuming of course it can be done with acceptable morbidity and mortality rates.[41]

Recent decades have introduced technological advancements that have rapidly transformed the capabilities of robotic surgical instruments and cameras, all of which have enabled more and more surgeons to successfully adopt minimally invasive techniques. However, as with all new technology, there is a required learning curve that is associated with these advancements.[19] The learning curve for the simplest laparoscopic gastrectomy—a distal gastrectomy for an early gastric cancer—has been estimated at approximately 60 to 90 cases, which is a daunting number for even a high-volume Western surgeon, who may perform fewer than 20 gastrectomies per year, the majority of which are for advanced cancers in obese, elderly patients.[18] For the more technically challenging minimally invasive total gastrectomy, the learning curve may be closer to 100 cases.[50] In contrast, for the surgeon with preestablished advanced laparoscopic skills, the learning curve required to achieve proficiency for either a laparoscopic or robotic gastrectomy for gastric cancer is likely to be much less steep (and thus require far fewer cases).[51,52] Furthermore, owing to the benefits of 3-dimensional imaging and articulating instruments, it is thought that robotic gastric surgery may have an easier learning curve than laparoscopic gastric surgery.[49]

SUMMARY

Minimally invasive surgical approaches to the treatment of gastric cancer have become increasingly more common with the publication of more and more data demonstrating the safety, feasibility, and oncologic equivalency of such approaches to conventional open gastrectomy. While appreciating the differences in gastric cancer incidence, patient stage at the time of diagnosis, and surgeon experience related to case volume in the East versus the West, additional larger studies from the West have begun to demonstrate outcomes similar to those published in studies from the East. Despite longer operative times, minimally invasive gastrectomy for gastric cancer is associated with less intraoperative blood loss, a decreased length of stay and time to oral feeds, and an improved quality of life.[53] Importantly, the decreased morbidity rate and the faster postoperative recovery associated with the minimally invasive approach increases the likelihood of patients receiving adjuvant treatment in a more timely fashion.[20,54] Ultimately, increased surgeon experience with minimally invasive techniques and larger, prospective randomized studies will continue to push the limits of minimally invasive surgery for the treatment of gastric cancer.

REFERENCES

1. Ervik FL M, Ferlay J, Mery L, et al. International agency for research on cancer. Cancer Today 2016. Available at: http://gco.iarc.fr/today. Accessed December 22, 2017.
2. Howlader NNA, Krapcho M, Miller D, et al, editors. SEER cancer statistics review, 1975-2014. St. Louis, (MO): National Cancer Institute; 2017. Available at: https://seer.cancer.gov/statfacts/html/stomach.html.
3. Anderson WF, Camargo MC, Fraumeni JF Jr, et al. Age-specific trends in incidence of noncardia gastric cancer in US adults. JAMA 2010;303(17):1723–8.
4. Japanese Gastric Cancer Association. Japanese gastric cancer treatment guidelines 2010 (ver. 3). Gastric Cancer 2011;14(2):113–23.
5. Cameron JL, Cameron AM. Current surgical therapy. 11th edition. Elsevier Saunders; 2014.
6. Kitano S, Iso Y, Moriyama M, et al. Laparoscopy-assisted Billroth I gastrectomy. Surg Laparosc Endosc 1994;4(2):146–8.
7. Cassidy MR, Gholami S, Strong VE. Minimally invasive surgery: the emerging role in gastric cancer. Surg Oncol Clin N Am 2017;26(2):193–212.
8. Kitano S, Shiraishi N, Fujii K, et al. A randomized controlled trial comparing open vs laparoscopy-assisted distal gastrectomy for the treatment of early gastric cancer: an interim report. Surgery 2002;131(1 Suppl):S306–11.
9. Huang KH, Lan YT, Fang WL, et al. Initial experience of robotic gastrectomy and comparison with open and laparoscopic gastrectomy for gastric cancer. J Gastrointest Surg 2012;16(7):1303–10.
10. Kim KM, An JY, Kim HI, et al. Major early complications following open, laparoscopic and robotic gastrectomy. Br J Surg 2012;99(12):1681–7.
11. Kunisaki C, Makino H, Takagawa R, et al. Efficacy of laparoscopy-assisted distal gastrectomy for gastric cancer in the elderly. Surg Endosc 2009;23(2):377–83.
12. Hwang SI, Kim HO, Yoo CH, et al. Laparoscopic-assisted distal gastrectomy versus open distal gastrectomy for advanced gastric cancer. Surg Endosc 2009;23(6):1252–8.
13. Kinoshita T, Uyama I, Terashima M, et al. Long-term outcomes of laparoscopic versus open surgery for clinical stage II/III gastric cancer: a multicenter cohort study in Japan (LOC-A Study). Ann Surg 2018. https://doi.org/10.1097/SLA.0000000000002768.
14. Cui M, Li Z, Xing J, et al. A prospective randomized clinical trial comparing D2 dissection in laparoscopic and open gastrectomy for gastric cancer. Med Oncol 2015;32(10):241.
15. Kim W, Kim HH, Han SU, et al. Decreased morbidity of laparoscopic distal gastrectomy compared with open distal gastrectomy for stage i gastric cancer: short-term outcomes from a multicenter randomized controlled trial (KLASS-01). Ann Surg 2016;263(1):28–35.
16. Aoyama T, Yoshikawa T, Hayashi T, et al. Randomized comparison of surgical stress and the nutritional status between laparoscopy-assisted and open distal gastrectomy for gastric cancer. Ann Surg Oncol 2014;21(6):1983–90.
17. Sakuramoto S, Yamashita K, Kikuchi S, et al. Laparoscopy versus open distal gastrectomy by expert surgeons for early gastric cancer in Japanese patients:

short-term clinical outcomes of a randomized clinical trial. Surg Endosc 2013; 27(5):1695–705.

18. Zhang X, Tanigawa N. Learning curve of laparoscopic surgery for gastric cancer, a laparoscopic distal gastrectomy-based analysis. Surg Endosc 2009;23(6): 1259–64.

19. Yoo CH, Kim HO, Hwang SI, et al. Short-term outcomes of laparoscopic-assisted distal gastrectomy for gastric cancer during a surgeon's learning curve period. Surg Endosc 2009;23(10):2250–7.

20. Kelly KJ, Selby L, Chou JF, et al. Laparoscopic versus open gastrectomy for gastric adenocarcinoma in the west: a case-control study. Ann Surg Oncol 2015;22(11):3590–6.

21. Strong VE, Devaud N, Allen PJ, et al. Laparoscopic versus open subtotal gastrectomy for adenocarcinoma: a case-control study. Ann Surg Oncol 2009;16(6): 1507–13.

22. Guzman EA, Pigazzi A, Lee B, et al. Totally laparoscopic gastric resection with extended lymphadenectomy for gastric adenocarcinoma. Ann Surg Oncol 2009;16(8):2218–23.

23. Huscher CG, Mingoli A, Sgarzini G, et al. Laparoscopic versus open subtotal gastrectomy for distal gastric cancer: five-year results of a randomized prospective trial. Ann Surg 2005;241(2):232–7.

24. Vinuela EF, Gonen M, Brennan MF, et al. Laparoscopic versus open distal gastrectomy for gastric cancer: a meta-analysis of randomized controlled trials and high-quality nonrandomized studies. Ann Surg 2012;255(3):446–56.

25. Zhang CD, Chen SC, Feng ZF, et al. Laparoscopic versus open gastrectomy for early gastric cancer in Asia: a meta-analysis. Surg Laparosc Endosc Percutan Tech 2013;23(4):365–77.

26. Kodera Y, Fujiwara M, Ohashi N, et al. Laparoscopic surgery for gastric cancer: a collective review with meta-analysis of randomized trials. J Am Coll Surg 2010; 211(5):677–86.

27. Ajani JA, Bentrem DJ, Besh S, et al. Gastric cancer, version 2.2013: featured updates to the NCCN guidelines. J Natl Compr Canc Netw 2013;11(5):531–46.

28. Bo T, Peiwu Y, Feng Q, et al. Laparoscopy-assisted vs. open total gastrectomy for advanced gastric cancer: long-term outcomes and technical aspects of a case-control study. J Gastrointest Surg 2013;17(7):1202–8.

29. Kim KH, Kim MC, Jung GJ, et al. Comparative analysis of five-year survival results of laparoscopy-assisted gastrectomy versus open gastrectomy for advanced gastric cancer: a case-control study using a propensity score method. Dig Surg 2012;29(2):165–71.

30. Fang C, Hua J, Li J, et al. Comparison of long-term results between laparoscopy-assisted gastrectomy and open gastrectomy with D2 lymphadenectomy for advanced gastric cancer. Am J Surg 2014;208(3):391–6.

31. Du XH, Li R, Chen L, et al. Laparoscopy-assisted D2 radical distal gastrectomy for advanced gastric cancer: initial experience. Chin Med J 2009;122(12): 1404–7.

32. Hur H, Jeon HM, Kim W. Laparoscopy-assisted distal gastrectomy with D2 lymphadenectomy for T2b advanced gastric cancers: three years' experience. J Surg Oncol 2008;98(7):515–9.

33. Cai J, Wei D, Gao CF, et al. A prospective randomized study comparing open versus laparoscopy-assisted D2 radical gastrectomy in advanced gastric cancer. Dig Surg 2011;28(5–6):331–7.

34. Hu Y, Huang C, Sun Y, et al. Morbidity and mortality of laparoscopic versus open D2 distal gastrectomy for advanced gastric cancer: a randomized controlled trial. J Clin Oncol 2016;34(12):1350–7.

35. Shi Y, Xu X, Zhao Y, et al. Short-term surgical outcomes of a randomized controlled trial comparing laparoscopic versus open gastrectomy with D2 lymph node dissection for advanced gastric cancer. Surg Endosc 2018;32(5):2427–33.

36. Lee JH. Ongoing surgical clinical trials on minimally invasive surgery for gastric cancer: Korea. Transl Gastroenterol Hepatol 2016;1:40.

37. Strand MS, Strong VE, Fields RC, et al. Gastrectomy for cancer: what are the benefits of a minimally invasive approach? Bull Am Coll Surg 2017;102(7):68–70.

38. Choi YY, Bae JM, An JY, et al. Laparoscopic gastrectomy for advanced gastric cancer: are the long-term results comparable with conventional open gastrectomy? A systematic review and meta-analysis. J Surg Oncol 2013;108(8):550–6.

39. Martinez-Ramos D, Miralles-Tena JM, Cuesta MA, et al. Laparoscopy versus open surgery for advanced and resectable gastric cancer: a meta-analysis. Rev Esp Enferm Dig 2011;103(3):133–41.

40. Chen K, Xu XW, Mou YP, et al. Systematic review and meta-analysis of laparoscopic and open gastrectomy for advanced gastric cancer. World J Surg Oncol 2013;11:182.

41. Songun I, Putter H, Kranenbarg EM, et al. Surgical treatment of gastric cancer: 15-year follow-up results of the randomised nationwide Dutch D1D2 trial. Lancet Oncol 2010;11(5):439–49.

42. Karpeh MS, Leon L, Klimstra D, et al. Lymph node staging in gastric cancer: is location more important than number? An analysis of 1,038 patients. Ann Surg 2000;232(3):362–71.

43. Coratti A, Fernandes E, Lombardi A, et al. Robot-assisted surgery for gastric carcinoma: five years follow-up and beyond: a single western center experience and long-term oncological outcomes. Eur J Surg Oncol 2015;41(8):1106–13.

44. Hashizume M, Sugimachi K. Robot-assisted gastric surgery. Surg Clin North Am 2003;83(6):1429–44.

45. Anderson C, Ellenhorn J, Hellan M, et al. Pilot series of robot-assisted laparoscopic subtotal gastrectomy with extended lymphadenectomy for gastric cancer. Surg Endosc 2007;21(9):1662–6.

46. Song J, Oh SJ, Kang WH, et al. Robot-assisted gastrectomy with lymph node dissection for gastric cancer: lessons learned from an initial 100 consecutive procedures. Ann Surg 2009;249(6):927–32.

47. Pan JH, Zhou H, Zhao XX, et al. Long-term oncological outcomes in robotic gastrectomy versus laparoscopic gastrectomy for gastric cancer: a meta-analysis. Surg Endosc 2017;31(10):4244–51.

48. Chen K, Pan Y, Zhang B, et al. Robotic versus laparoscopic Gastrectomy for gastric cancer: a systematic review and updated meta-analysis. BMC Surg 2017;17(1):93.

49. Quijano Y, Vicente E, Ielpo B, et al. Full robot-assisted gastrectomy: surgical technique and preliminary experience from a single center. J Robot Surg 2016;10(4):297–306.

50. Jung DH, Son SY, Park YS, et al. The learning curve associated with laparoscopic total gastrectomy. Gastric Cancer 2016;19(1):264–72.

51. Park SS, Kim MC, Park MS, et al. Rapid adaptation of robotic gastrectomy for gastric cancer by experienced laparoscopic surgeons. Surg Endosc 2012;26(1):60–7.

52. Huang KH, Lan YT, Fang WL, et al. Comparison of the operative outcomes and learning curves between laparoscopic and robotic gastrectomy for gastric cancer. PLoS One 2014;9(10):e111499.
53. Kim YW, Baik YH, Yun YH, et al. Improved quality of life outcomes after laparoscopy-assisted distal gastrectomy for early gastric cancer: results of a prospective randomized clinical trial. Ann Surg 2008;248(5):721–7.
54. Russo A, Strong VE. Minimally invasive surgery for gastric cancer in USA: current status and future perspectives. Transl Gastroenterol Hepatol 2017;2:38.
55. Kim MC, Kim KH, Kim HH, et al. Comparison of laparoscopy-assisted by conventional open distal gastrectomy and extraperigastric lymph node dissection in early gastric cancer. J Surg Oncol 2005;91(1):90–4.
56. Lee SE, Kim YW, Lee JH, et al. Developing an institutional protocol guideline for laparoscopy-assisted distal gastrectomy. Ann Surg Oncol 2009;16(8):2231–6.
57. Suda K, Man IM, Ishida Y, et al. Potential advantages of robotic radical gastrectomy for gastric adenocarcinoma in comparison with conventional laparoscopic approach: a single institutional retrospective comparative cohort study. Surg Endosc 2015;29(3):673–85.
58. Lee JH, Yom CK, Han HS. Comparison of long-term outcomes of laparoscopy-assisted and open distal gastrectomy for early gastric cancer. Surg Endosc 2009;23(8):1759–63.
59. Hayashi H, Ochiai T, Shimada H, et al. Prospective randomized study of open versus laparoscopy-assisted distal gastrectomy with extraperigastric lymph node dissection for early gastric cancer. Surg Endosc 2005;19(9):1172–6.
60. Kim HH, Hyung WJ, Cho GS, et al. Morbidity and mortality of laparoscopic gastrectomy versus open gastrectomy for gastric cancer: an interim report–a phase III multicenter, prospective, randomized trial (KLASS trial). Ann Surg 2010;251(3):417–20.
61. Takiguchi S, Fujiwara Y, Yamasaki M, et al. Laparoscopy-assisted distal gastrectomy versus open distal gastrectomy. A prospective randomized single-blind study. World J Surg 2013;37(10):2379–86.

Minimally Invasive Primary Liver Cancer Surgery

Forat Swaid, MD*, David A. Geller, MD

KEYWORDS

- Hepato-cellular carcinoma • Laparoscopic liver resection • Overall survival

KEY POINTS

- Liver resection is a valuable treatment option for carefully selected patients with hepato-cellular carcinoma (HCC).
- Early concerns with incorporating laparoscopy into liver surgery have been invalidated.
- In general, patients undergoing laparoscopic liver resection (LLR) had less blood loss, fewer transfusions, less postoperative morbidity, and shorter lengths of stay compared with open liver resections (OLR) cases.
- The 5-year overall survival for patients undergoing LLR for HCC ranged from 50% to 90%, and not a single study showed worse 5-year overall survival comparing LLR with OLR.

INTRODUCTION

Hepatocellular carcinoma (HCC) is the most common primary malignancy of the liver.[1] It has a high incidence (especially in Asia) with more than 700,000 new cases each year globally and is considered the sixth most common type of cancer worldwide and the third leading cause of cancer-related death.[2] Treatment options with curative intent include liver transplantation, resection, and ablation. Liver transplantation is considered an optimal treatment, because it is associated with the lowest recurrence rates, and it also addresses the background liver cirrhosis, which exists in more than 80% of patients with HCC.[2] However, the incidence of HCC is increasing, and there is a constant donor organ shortage, both factors making liver transplantation not a feasible treatment option for many patients.[3]

Liver resection is an excellent treatment option for selected patients with HCC.[4] However, in cirrhotic patients, resection can be associated with potential complications, for example, worsening ascites and liver failure.[5] Therefore, cirrhotic patients

Disclosure Statement: The authors have no conflicts of interest and have nothing to disclose.
Department of Surgery, Division of Hepatobiliary and Pancreatic Surgery, UPMC Liver Cancer Center, University of Pittsburgh Medical Center, 3471 Fifth Avenue, Suite 300, Pittsburgh, PA 15213, USA
* Corresponding author.
E-mail address: foratola@gmail.com

should be carefully selected when considering resection, and the patients with more advanced cirrhosis are potentially better served with liver transplantation.

For decades, open compared with laparoscopic surgery has been considered as being "more suitable" for liver resections. Early concerns with incorporating laparoscopy into liver surgery included the risk of CO_2 embolization in the case of injury of a hepatic vein. However, this complication was shown to occur only rarely.[6,7] In addition, the concern of excessive bleeding during laparoscopic liver resection (LLR), attributed to the inability to apply manual compression of bleeding vessels, was also invalidated. In fact, most reports show that LLR is associated with less blood loss and lower transfusion needs. Similar to other fields in surgery, proponents of LLR had to first provide evidence that it is not inferior to the standard open liver resections (OLR), and then they had to show that it has some advantages over the established open approach.[8]

The first report on LLR appeared in 1992,[9] followed by the first LLR for the indication of HCC by Hashizume and colleagues[10] in 1995. Gradually thereafter, reports and case series with increasing numbers of LLR emerged. With marked advancements in technology, as well as improvements in the understanding of liver anatomy and better preoperative radiologic imaging, a paradigm shift came about with tremendous growth in the number of LLR.

Following these early reports, 2 international LLR consensus conferences convened, the first in Louisville, Kentucky in 2008,[11] and the second in Morioka, Japan in 2014.[12] The first conference stated that minor LLRs are safe and should be a standard practice. The results from the Second International Consensus Conference were published with recommendations given by a 9-member independent jury and an expert panel of surgeons. Major LLR was considered an innovative procedure, still in an exploration or learning phase, and with incompletely defined risks. The recommendations of these consensus conferences were based on a relatively large number of reports, including series with propensity score matching as well as meta-analyses, almost all of which showing not only noninferiority of LLR compared with OLR but also superiority of LLR in several parameters, as discussed in detail later.

LLR is implemented today in virtually all types of liver diseases and conditions, including laparoscopic live donor hepatectomies. In 2009, Nguyen and colleagues[13] published a world literature review that included 127 articles on LLR, accounting for 2804 patients. Fifty percent of LLRs were for malignant tumors, and 75% were performed totally laparoscopically, with the most commonly performed procedure being wedge resection or segmentectomy (45%). Mortality was 9 of 2804 patients (0.3%), and morbidity was 10.5%, with no intraoperative deaths reported. For cancer resections, negative surgical margins were achieved in 82% to 100% of patients in the reported series. The 5-year overall survival (OS) and disease-free survival (DFS) rates after LLR for HCC were 50% to 75% and 31% to 38.2%, respectively. The large numbers reported in this highly sited review were important for the demonstration of the safety and feasibility of LLR.

Among primary liver cancer, the focus of this article is on LLR for HCC. The different parameters reported in the literature comparing LLR to OLR are discussed in detail with reference to key reports addressing each parameter. **Table 1** provides an OS in 16 studies and 3 meta-analysis comparing 5-year OS of LLR versus OLR in matched patients. The 5-year OS ranged from 50% to 90% in LLR, and not a single study showed worse 5-year OS comparing LLR to OLR. **Table 2** summarizes the perioperative outcomes comparing LLR to OLR. In general, patients undergoing LLR had less blood loss, fewer transfusions, less postoperative morbidity, and shorter length of stay (LOS) compared with OLR cases.

Table 1
Studies with 5-y survival comparison between laparoscopic liver resection and open liver resection

Reference, y	No. of Patients LLR/OLR	Country	Journal	5-y Survival, %		Statistical Significance
				LLR	OLR	
Sotiropoulos et al,[14] 2017[a]	2112/3019	Greece	*Updates Surg*	HR = 0.97 (95% CI 0.82–1.14)		NS
Cheung et al,[15] 2016	110/330	Hong Kong	*Ann Surg*	52	48	NS
Chang et al,[16] 2016	30/30	Singapore	*Ann Acad Med Singapore*	59	65	NS
Takahara et al,[17] 2015	387/387	Japan	*J Hepatobiliary Pancreat Sci*	77	71	NS
Kim et al,[18] 2014	29/29	Korea	*Surg Endosc*	92	88	NS
Yin et al,[19] 2013[a]	485/753	China	*Ann Surg Oncol*	HR = 0.99 (95% CI 0.74–1.33)		NS
Cheung et al,[20] 2013	32/64	China	*Ann Surg*	77	57	NS
Ker et al,[21] 2011	116/208	Taiwan	*Int J Hepatol*	62	72	NS
Truant et al,[22] 2011	35/53	France	*Surg Endosc*	70	46	NS
Zhou et al,[23] 2011[a]	213/281	China	*Dig Dis Sci*	HR = 1.64 (95% CI 0.92–2.93)		NS
Fancellu et al,[24] 2011[a]	227/363	Italy	*J Surg Res*	63	56	NS
Lee et al,[25] 2011	33/50	China	*World J Surg*	76	76	NS
Hu et al,[26] 2011	30/30	China	*World J Gastroenterol*	50	53	NS
Tranchart et al,[27] 2010	42/42	France	*Surg Endosc*	60	47	NS
Sarpel et al,[28] 2009	20/56	USA	*Ann Surg Oncol*	95	75	NS
Endo et al,[29] 2009	10/11	Japan	*Surg Laparosc Endosc Percutan Tech*	57	48	NS
Cai et al,[30] 2008	31/31	China	*Surg Endosc*	50	51	NS
Kaneko et al,[31] 2005	30/28	Japan	*Am J Surg*	61	62	NS
Shimada et al,[32] 2001	17/38	Japan	*Surg Endosc*	50	38	NS

Abbreviations: HR, hazard ratio; NS, nonsignificant.
[a] Meta-analyses.

Table 2
Studies with comparison of intraoperative and postoperative outcomes between laparoscopic liver resection and open liver resection

Reference, y	No. of Patients LLR/OLR	Less Blood Loss	Fewer Transfusions	Shorter OR Time	Less Overall Morbidity	Shorter LOS	Higher R0 Rate
Chang et al,[16] 2019	30/30	LLR	N/A	N/A	N/A	LLR	Equivalent
Takahara et al,[17] 2015	387/387	LLR	LLR	OLR	LLR	LLR	N/A
Chen et al,[33] 2015	281/547	LLR	LLR	Equivalent	N/A	LLR	LLR
Cheung et al,[15] 2016	110/330	LLR	Equivalent	LLR	Equivalent	LLR	N/A
Komatsu et al,[34] 2016	38/38	Equivalent	Equivalent	OLR	LLR	Equivalent	Equivalent
Xu et al,[69]	32/32	LLR	Equivalent	OLR	Equivalent	Equivalent	N/A
Sotiropoulos et al,[14] 2017[a]	2112/3019	LLR	LLR	Equivalent	LLR	LLR	LLR
Chen et al,[35] 2017	225/291	LLR	LLR	Minor resections: LLR Major resections: OLR	Equivalent	LLR	N/A
Xiong et al,[36] 2012	234/316	LLR	LLR	Equivalent	LLR	LLR	Equivalent
Li et al,[37] 2012[a]	244/383	LLR	LLR	Equivalent	LLR	LLR	Equivalent
Mizuguchi et al,[38] 2011[a]	232/253	LLR	N/A	Equivalent	LLR	LLR	N/A
Yin et al,[19] 2013[a]	485/753	LLR	LLR	Equivalent	LLR	LLR	Equivalent
Zhou et al,[23] 2011[a]	213/281	LLR	LLR	Equivalent	LLR	LLR	Equivalent
Fancellu et al,[24] 2011[a]	227/363	LLR	LLR	Equivalent	LLR	LLR	LLR

[a] Meta-analyses.

SURGICAL MARGINS

Achieving negative resection margins is the mainstay of oncologic surgery and is associated with improved survival. Chang and colleagues[16] reported that LLR achieved negative resection margins in 97% of patients, similar to OLR. Furthermore, several reports showed that LLR was associated with wider resection margins compared with OLR.[14,33] In general, most of the case-match series showed comparable resection margins, and no study showed a lower R0 resection rate for LLR compared with OLR. Achieving similar rates of negative margins explains the reported similar local recurrence rates between LLR and OLR in studies reporting on this important outcome parameter.[14,16]

BLOOD LOSS AND NEED FOR TRANSFUSION

Perhaps the most constant finding in most reports comparing LLR with OLR is that LLR is associated with less intraoperative blood loss, and less transfusion requirements.[14–17,19,23,24,33,35–37,39–41] These findings leave little doubt that this is one parameter whereby LLR may be superior to OLR, thus eliminating early concerns of "loss of control" of bleeding during laparoscopic parenchymal transection. Chen and colleagues[35] showed that this is true not only for minor but also for major laparoscopic resections compared with an open approach.

One contributing factor to these findings may be the pneumoperitoneum during LLR. The standard pneumoperitoneum pressure is set to 12 mm Hg, considerably higher than the average central venous pressure during parenchymal transection, which is commonly intentionally decreased by the anesthesiologists to 5 mm Hg or less. This pressure difference occludes small vein branches at the cut surface of the liver that usually ooze slowly but continuously during OLR.[42–45] An additional explanation for the lower blood loss with LLR may be the magnification provided by the laparoscope, facilitating recognition and precise control of small bleeding vessels. Furthermore, the advanced modern laparoscopic instruments have excellent hemostatic capabilities.[46] The new generation of power-driven stapling devices potentially allows for smoother and safer stapling of intrahepatic structures, thus potentially contributing to improved hemostasis.[47,48] Achieving better hemostasis is particularly important for oncologic resections, because several studies have shown that excessive blood loss and transfusion requirements are associated with worse short- and long-term outcomes and can have a negative impact on prognosis.[49,50]

OPERATIVE TIME

In contrast to blood loss, whereby there is general agreement in the literature about the superiority of LLR over OLR, reports on operative time are less homogeneous.

Cheung and colleagues[15] reported a shorter operation time with LLR. Chen and colleagues[35] reached a similar conclusion, but only in patients undergoing minor LLR. For major OLR, LLR was associated with significantly longer operative time. These findings can be explained by the more established techniques and experience with minor LLRs, which usually do not involve lengthy liver mobilizations and gaining vascular control, steps that require advanced laparoscopic skills. In minor LLR, the resections are usually straightforward and are done with energy devices such as ultrasonic shears, and minimal time is spent on making or closing the incisions, as compared with OLR. Conversely, major LLRs are still exploratory techniques; experience is more limited, and they require major manipulations of the liver that can be technically challenging when performed laparoscopically. Although some reports showed no significant difference in operative time between LLR and OLR,[14] others showed that operative time in LLR was significantly longer.[17] Therefore, because operative time is a parameter dependent on surgical skills, training, experience, case volume, and learning curve, operative time is reported heterogeneously among the different groups without one conclusive result.

LENGTH OF STAY AND OVERALL POSTOPERATIVE MORBIDITY

In concordance with data from other fields of abdominal surgery, LLR is almost unanimously associated with significantly shorter hospitalization as compared with OLR. In a multi-institutional Japanese study with propensity score matching, Takahara and colleagues[17] reported a shorter hospital stay for patients undergoing LLR for HCC. Several other major reports and analyses confirmed this trend.[14–16,33,35,39] Shorter LOS has been shown to be true for both minor and major LLRs, when evaluated separately.[35] It is well established that the smaller incisions and lesser degree of trauma to the abdominal wall during laparoscopic abdominal surgery lead to less pain, better mobility, fewer atelectasis and pulmonary complications,[51,52] fewer wound infections, and less wound dehiscence, all of which contribute to quicker recovery and shorter hospitalization. LLRs are no exception to this rule. The incisions used for OLR are usually large subcostal or hockey stick incisions that cut through the abdominal wall musculature and cause painful breathing postoperatively. Furthermore, the significant retraction applied to the lower ribs during OLR contributes to the discomfort associated with these incisions. Because laparoscopy eliminates these factors, it is not surprising to see the lower rates of pain and quicker recovery associated with LLR, leading to shorter LOS.

Even in major laparoscopic resections, whereby an incision is needed for specimen retrieval, these extraction incisions are usually created in the lower abdomen, generally leading to lower pain and fewer pulmonary complications. One commonly used extraction incision in laparoscopic resections is the Pfannenstiel incision, which is generally associated with excellent cosmetic results and low morbidity, especially in regards to low-incisional hernia rates, reported to range between 0% and 2%.[53,54] Although most reports reviewed showed lower overall complication rates in LLR than in OLR,[17,33,39] some showed the overall complication rates between the 2 groups were not significantly different.[15,35]

DISEASE-FREE AND OVERALL SURVIVAL

For LLR to become a viable option for treating HCC, it was critical to demonstrate that it is at least noninferior to OLR in oncologic outcomes. Indeed, most reports in the literature show comparable OS and DFS rates between LLR and OLR.[14,16,17,39] Not only was LLR established as an oncologically noninferior operation compared with OLR but also some investigators demonstrated superior results with LLR. Chen and colleagues[33] reported better 5-year survival rate with LLR compared with OLR (relative risk = 1.28, 95% confidence interval [CI] 1.01–1.62, $P = .04$).[33]

Cheung and colleagues[15] reported statistically significant 1-, 3-, and 5-year OS differences in favor of LLR over OLR, with reported rates of 98.9%, 89.8%, and 83.7%, respectively, in the LLR group, and 94%, 79.3%, and 67.4%, respectively, in the OLR group ($P = .033$).[15] The 1-, 3-, and 5-year DFS rates were also better for the LLR group, at 87.7%, 65.8%, and 52.2%, respectively, in the LLR group, and 75.2%, 56.3%, and 47.9%, respectively, in the OLR group ($P = .141$). The 2 groups had similar cancer staging on final pathology. When patients were broken into groups based on their HCC stage, the OS and DFS differences were significant in patients with stage II HCC, but not in patients with stage I HCC (5-year DFS stage II HCC: 54.2% vs

40.1% of LLR vs OLR, $P = .045$). The investigators attributed these results, favoring LLR over OLR, to 2 factors: first, less blood loss in the LLR group; blood loss is known to be a risk factor for HCC recurrence.[55] Second, in contrast to significant mobilization and tissue manipulation before and during parenchymal transection for the OLR, the laparoscopic resections were performed using the anterior approach, with parenchymal transection taking place before any significant mobilization. Thus a no-touch" technique is performed, which may be associated with improved oncologic outcomes.[56,57]

Cipriani and colleagues[58] showed that the overall recurrence-free survival (RFS) was shorter in patients with advanced cirrhosis undergoing LLR for HCC, compared with patients with early cirrhosis undergoing LLR (43 vs 55 months, respectively, $P = .034$). However, when examined carefully, the rate of recurrence at the resection margin or in the same segment was not different between the 2 groups. Hence, the higher recurrence rate in advanced cirrhotic livers probably reflects the carcinogenic effect of advanced cirrhosis rather than an impact of an LLR approach.[59,60]

RESECTIONS IN CIRRHOTIC PATIENTS

Nearly 80% of HCC develop in cirrhotic livers. Hepatectomy in cirrhotic patients is associated with higher complication rates, including infection, pleural effusion, ascites decompensation, and liver failure,[61-63] thus deterring many surgeons from performing liver resections in patients with advanced cirrhosis. Contributing factors to the increased complexity of liver resections in cirrhotic patients include firm and friable liver parenchyma, portal hypertension, and thrombocytopenia, factors that make hemostasis more challenging. Furthermore, it is widely reported that liver resections in cirrhotic patients are associated with a relatively high hospital mortality of 1% to 4%, even at high-volume centers.[64-66] Therefore, LLR in cirrhotic patients is conceptually perceived as being risky, and in many centers, Child–Pugh B patients are precluded from laparoscopic resections.

However, the concept that LLR is too risky in patients with advanced cirrhosis has been challenged. Cipriani and colleagues[58] compared laparoscopic resections in early well-compensated Child–Pugh A patients with laparoscopic resections in more advanced, decompensated, Child–Pugh B patients. There was no significant difference between the 2 groups regarding blood loss, blood transfusions, operative time, Pringle maneuver duration, overall morbidity, and postoperative mortality. Even liver-specific complications, such as ascites decompensation and postoperative liver failure, were similar between the 2 groups. RFS in Child–Pugh B cirrhotics was significantly shorter than in Child–Pugh A patients, but OS was not significantly different between the 2 groups.

These results suggest that laparoscopy may offer a protective effect with regard to postoperative liver failure and ascites, even in Child–Pugh B patients. A possible explanation could be that cirrhotics with portal hypertension have extensive collateral blood vessels in the abdominal wall. During open surgery, much of this collateral circulation is disrupted by the large abdominal incision. Disruption of this collateral circulation contribute to increased ascites and liver decompensation postoperatively. In LLR, this factor is minimized, possibly explaining the relatively good tolerance and low rate of decompensation following surgery, even in advanced cirrhosis.[27,62,67] The safety and possible advantages of LLR in cirrhotic patients have been demonstrated in reports[15,33] comparing OLR with LLR. In these reports, LLR has been associated with lower incidence of ascites decompensation and liver failure as mentioned above.[62,68] This "protective" effect of laparoscopy may be more prominent in major hepatectomies. Xu and colleagues[69] compared patients undergoing major liver resections either laparoscopically or via open surgery. The LLR group had a significantly longer operative time (255 vs 200 minutes, $P<.001$). The blood loss and transfusion requirement were comparable. The rate of overall postoperative complications did not differ between groups, whereas the incidence of ascites in the LLR group was significantly less (9.4 vs 31.3%, $P = .030$). The oncologic outcomes between the 2 groups were comparable with regard to OS and DFS. Similarly, Komatsu and colleagues[34] also compared patients undergoing open or laparoscopic major hepatectomies. There were no significant differences in blood loss, blood transfusion rate, OS, or DFS between the 2 groups. The overall complication rates were significantly higher in the OLR group, with the most common complications being surgical site infections, ascites decompensation, and liver failure.

In a recent report, Beard and colleagues[70] compared LLR for HCC in 80 patients with early (Child's A) cirrhosis to 26 patients with advanced cirrhosis (20 Child's B and 6 Child's C). There were no significant differences between the 2 patient groups in terms of blood loss, conversion, negative margin rates, LOS, perioperative complications, 30-day mortality, and 90-day mortality. Although a trend toward longer survival in patients with Child's A cirrhosis was noted, this did not reach statistical significance (50 vs 21 months, $P = .077$).

HEPATOCELLULAR CARCINOMA LOCATED IN "DIFFICULT SEGMENTS"

With increasing experience, the limits of LLR are being constantly pushed. In addition to performing major hepatectomies laparoscopically, which became standard in some centers, lesions in difficult, inaccessible parts of the posterior-superior liver are being resected laparoscopically in experienced hands. Guro and colleagues[71] compared LLR with OLR for HCC located in segments 7 and 8. LLR was associated with less blood loss and shorter hospital stay. There were no statistically significant differences between the 2 groups in operative time, postoperative complications, rate of negative resection margins, and the 3-year OS and DFS rates.

ROBOTIC RESECTIONS

After the technical feasibility and oncologic safety of LLR for HCC have been demonstrated, robotic liver resections are now on the increase. The flexibility and versatility given by the robotic approach have the potential for making larger and posteriorly located tumors more easily accessible to minimally invasive resection. In one report, Lai and Tang[72] compared the long-term oncologic outcomes of robotic and laparoscopic hepatectomy for HCC. The rate of major resections and resections for lesions in posterior-superior segments was significantly higher in the robotic group compared with the laparoscopic group (27% vs 2.9%, and 29% vs 0%, respectively). Operative time was significantly longer in the robotic group. There was no significant difference in blood loss, morbidity, mortality, R0 resection, OS, and DFS rates.

In 2014, Tsung and colleagues[73] published a matched comparison between patients undergoing robotic (n = 57) and laparoscopic (n = 114) liver resections. Although this series included patients with not only HCC, it was the largest published work with such a comparison. There were no significant differences between the 2 groups in terms of blood loss, rate of negative margins, postoperative peak bilirubin levels, intensive care unit admission rate, LOS, and 90-day mortality. One disadvantage of the robotic resections was that they were associated with a significantly longer operative time, and overall room time, when compared with laparoscopic resections (253 vs 199 minutes, and 342 vs 262 minutes, respectively). However, in the robotic group, significantly more major resections were performed in a purely minimally invasive approach, compared with the laparoscopic resections, which were associated with higher rates of hand-port or hybrid assistance.

ADDITIONAL BENEFITS OF LAPAROSCOPIC LIVER RESECTION

Because HCC usually occurs in cirrhotic livers, recurrence in the remaining liver is not uncommon after resections. Therefore, many patients need repeat resections. It is well established that LLR make future resections easier, because of less adhesions associated with OLR.[74,75] Some reports have also shown that redo LLRs are associated with better short-term outcomes.[67,76–78] In addition, in general, laparoscopic resections are associated with improved cosmetic results, lower rates of incisional hernias, and quicker return to work.

RANDOMIZED CLINICAL TRIAL OF LAPAROSCOPIC LIVER RESECTION VERSUS OPEN LIVER RESECTION FOR HEPATOCELLULAR CARCINOMA

A recent randomized clinical trial of LLR versus OLR for solitary HCC less than 5 cm in Child's A cirrhotics with peripheral segment tumors (II–VI) was performed.[79] The patients were well matched for age, gender, American Society of Anesthesiologists score, body mass index, hepatitis C virus, tumor location, tumor size (3.3 cm), and alpha-fetoprotein levels. The LLR group had less operating room (OR) time (120 vs 147 min, $P<.001$), shorter LOS (2.4 vs 4.3 days, $P<.001$), less intravenous (IV) narcotic use (1.0 vs 2.8 days, $P = .0001$), and shorter time to regular diet versus OLR. There was no difference in estimated blood loss, packed red blood cells treatment, R0 rate, overall complications, or 1- (88%, 84%) and 3-year (59%, 54%) DFS between groups.

SUMMARY

In summary, LLR has been performed in more than 10,000 patients worldwide. Comparable oncologic outcomes (R0 rate, 5-year DFS, and 5-year OS) have been reported for LLR for HCC compared with OLR using case controls, propensity score matching, and meta-analyses. A small randomized clinical trial for HCC showed shorter OR time, LOS, IV narcotic use, and time to regular diet in the minimally invasive surgery (MIS) group with similar 1- and 3-year DFS. Although most reports of LLR are in Child's A cirrhotic patients, a few studies have shown the feasibility of LLR in selected Child's B/C patients, and further studies will need to define which patients with advanced cirrhosis and HCC are suitable for an MIS approach.

REFERENCES

1. Torre LA, Bray F, Siegel RL, et al. Global cancer statistics, 2012. CA Cancer J Clin 2015;65:87–108.
2. Llovet JM, Burroughs A, Bruix J. Hepatocellular carcinoma. Lancet 2003;362: 1907–17.
3. Bruix J, Sherman M. Management of hepatocellular car- cinoma: an update. Hepatology 2011;53(3):1020–2.
4. Forner A, Reig ME, de Lope CR, et al. Current strategy for staging and treatment: the BCLC update and future prospects. Semin Liver Dis 2010;30:61–74.
5. Ishizawa T, Hasegawa K, Kokudo N, et al. Risk factors and manage- ment of ascites after liver resection to treat hepatocellular carcinoma. Arch Surg 2009;144: 46–51.

6. Tang CN, Tsui KK, Ha JP, et al. A single-centre experience of 40 laparoscopic liver resections. Hong Kong Med J 2006;12:419–25.

7. Bazin JE, Gillart T, Rasson P, et al. Haemodynamic conditions enhancing gas embolism after venous injury during laparoscopy: a study in pigs. Br J Anaesth 1997;78:570–5.

8. Wakabayashi G, Cherqui D, Geller DA, et al. Laparoscopic hepatectomy is theoretically better than open hepatectomy: preparing for the 2nd international consensus confer- ence on laparoscopic liver resection. J Hepatobiliary Pancreat Sci 2014;21:723–31.

9. Gagner M, Rheault M, Dubuc J. Laparoscopic partial hepatectomy for liver tumor. Surg Endosc 1992;6(2):99.

10. Hashizume M, Takenaka K, Yanaga K, et al. Laparoscopic hepatic resection for hepatocellular carcinoma. Surg Endosc 1995;9(12):1289–91.

11. Buell JF, Cherqui D, Geller DA, et al. The international position on laparoscopic liver surgery: The Louisville Statement, 2008. Ann Surg 2009;250:825–30.

12. Wakabayashi G, Cherqui D, Geller DA, et al. Recommendations for laparoscopic liver resection: a report from the second international consensus conference held in Morioka. Ann Surg 2015;261:619–29.

13. Nguyen KT, Gamblin TC, Geller DA. World review of laparoscopic liver resection-2,804 patients. Ann Surg 2009;250(5):831–41.

14. Sotiropoulos GC, Prodromidou A, Kostakis ID, et al. Meta-analysis of laparoscopic vs open liver resection for hepatocellular carcinoma. Updates Surg 2017;69:291.

15. Cheung TT, Dai WC, Tsang SH, et al. Pure laparoscopic hepatectomy versus open hepatectomy for hepatocellular carcinoma in 110 patients with liver cirrhosis: a propensity analysis at a single center. Ann Surg 2016;264(4):612–20.

16. Chang SK, Tay CW, Shen L, et al. Long-term oncological safety of minimally invasive hepatectomy in patients with hepatocellular carcinoma: a case-control study. Ann Acad Med Singapore 2016;45(3):91–7.

17. Takahara T, Wakabayashi G, Beppu T, et al. Long-term and perioperative outcomes of laparoscopic versus open liver resection for hepatocellular carcinoma with propensity score matching: a multi-institutional Japanese study. J Hepatobiliary Pancreat Sci 2015;22:721–7.

18. Kim H, Suh KS, Lee KW, et al. Long-term outcome of laparoscopic versus open liver resection for hepatocellular carcinoma: a case-controlled study with propensity score matching. Surg Endosc 2014;28:950–60.

19. Yin Z, Fan X, Ye H, et al. Short- and long-term outcomes after laparoscopic and open hepatectomy for hepatocel- lular carcinoma: a global systematic review and meta-analysis. Ann Surg Oncol 2013;20(4):1203–15.

20. Cheung TT, Poon RT, Yuen WK, et al. Long-term survival analysis of pure laparoscopic versus open hepatectomy for hepatocellular carcinoma in patients with cirrhosis: a single-center experience. Ann Surg 2013;257(3):506–11.

21. Ker CG, Chen JS, Kuo KK, et al. Liver surgery for hepatocellular carcinoma: laparoscopic versus open approach. Int J Hepatol 2011;2011:596792.

22. Truant S, Bouras AF, Hebbar M, et al. Laparoscopic resection vs. open liver resection for peripheral hepatocellular carcinoma in patients with chronic liver disease: a case-matched study. Surg Endosc 2011;25:3668–77.

23. Zhou YM, Shao WY, Zhao YF, et al. Meta- analysis of laparoscopic versus open resection for hepatocellular carcinoma. Dig Dis Sci 2011;56(7):1937–43.

24. Fancellu A, Rosman AS, Sanna V, et al. Meta-analysis of trials comparing minimally- invasive and open liver resections for hepatocellular carcinoma. J Surg Res 2011;171(1):e33–45.

25. Lee KF, Chong CN, Wong J, et al. Long-term results of laparoscopic hepatectomy versus open hepatectomy for hepatocellular carcinoma: a case-matched analysis. World J Surg 2011;35:2268–74.

26. Hu BS, Chen K, Tan HM, et al. Comparison of laparoscopic vs open liver lobectomy (segmentectomy) for hepatocellular carcinoma. World J Gastroenterol 2011; 17:4725–8.

27. Tranchart H, Di Giuro G, Lainas P, et al. Laparoscopic resection for hepatocellular carcinoma: a matched-pair comparative study. Surg Endosc 2010;24:1170–6.

28. Sarpel U, Hefti MM, Wisnievsky JP, et al. Outcome for patients treated with laparoscopic versus open resection of hepatocellular carcinoma: case-matched analysis. Ann Surg Oncol 2009;16(6):1572–7.

29. Endo Y, Ohta M, Sasaki A, et al. A comparative study of the long-term outcomes after laparoscopy-assisted and open left lateral hepatectomy for hepatocellular carcinoma. Surg Laparosc Endosc Percutan Tech 2009;19(5):e171–4.

30. Cai XJ, Yang J, Yu H, et al. Clinical study of laparoscopic versus open hepatectomy for malignant liver tumors. Surg Endosc 2008;22(11):2350–6.

31. Kaneko H, Takagi S, Otsuka Y, et al. Laparoscopic liver resection of hepatocellular carcinoma. Am J Surg 2005;189(2):190–4.

32. Shimada M, Hashizume M, Maehara S, et al. Laparoscopic hepatectomy for hepatocellular carcinoma. Surg Endosc 2001;15(6):541–4.

33. Chen J, Bai T, Zhang Y, et al. The safety and efficacy of laparoscopic and open hepatectomy in hepatocellular carcinoma patients with liver cirrhosis: a systematic review. Int J Clin Exp Med 2015;8(11):20679–89.

34. Komatsu S, Brustia R, Goumard C, et al. Laparoscopic versus open major hepatectomy for hepatocellular carcinoma: a matched pair analysis. Surg Endosc 2016;30:1965.

35. Chen J, Li H, Liu F, et al. Surgical outcomes of laparoscopic versus open liver resection for hepatocellular carcinoma for various resection extent. Medicine 2017;96(12):e6460.

36. Xiong JJ, Altaf K, Javed MA, et al. Meta-analysis of laparoscopic vs open liver resection for hepatocellular carcinoma. World J Gastroenterol 2012;18(45): 6657–68.

37. Li N, Wu YR, Wu B, et al. Surgical and oncologic outcomes following laparoscopic versus open liver resection for hepatocellular carcinoma: a meta-analysis. Hepatol Res 2012;42(1):51–9.

38. Mizuguchi T, Kawamoto M, Meguro M, et al. Laparoscopic hepatectomy: a systematic review, meta-analysis, and power analysis. Surg Today 2011;41(1):39–47.

39. Han DH, Choi SH, Park EJ, et al. Surgical outcomes after laparoscopic or robotic liver resection in hepatocellular carcinoma: a propensity-score matched analysis with conventional open liver resection. Int J Med Robot 2016;12:735–42.

40. Mirnezami R, Mirnezami AH, Chandrakumaran K, et al. Short- and long- term outcomes after laparoscopic and open hepatic resection: systematic review and meta-analysis. HPB (Oxford) 2011;13(5):295–308.

41. Parks KR, Kuo YH, Davis JM, et al. Laparoscopic versus open liver resection: a meta-analysis of long-term out- come. HPB (Oxford) 2014;16(2):109–18.

42. Belli G, Fantini C, D'Agostino A, et al. Laparoscopic liver resection without a Pringle maneuver for HCC in cirrhotic patients. Chir Ital 2005;57:15–25 [in Italian].

43. Jayaraman S, Khakhar A, Yang H, et al. The association between central venous pressure, pneumoperitoneum, and venous carbon dioxide embolism in laparoscopic hepatectomy. Surg Endosc 2009;23:2369–73.
44. Cherqui D, Husson E, Hammoud R, et al. Laparoscopic liver resections: a feasibility study in 30 patients. Ann Surg 2000;232:753–62.
45. Otsuka Y, Katagiri T, Ishii J, et al. Gasembolisminlaparoscopichepatectomy: what is the optimal pneumoperitoneal pressure for laparoscopic major hep- atectomy? J Hepatobiliary Pancreat Sci 2013;20:137–40.
46. Chiappa A, Bertani E, Biffi R, et al. Effectiveness of LigaSure diathermy coagulation in liver surgery. Surg Technol Int 2008;17:33–8.
47. Gayet B, Cavaliere D, Vibert E, et al. Totally laparoscopic right hepatectomy. Am J Surg 2007;194:685–9.
48. Gumbs AA, Gayet B. Totally laparoscopic left hepatectomy. Surg Endosc 2007; 21:1221.
49. Jarnagin WR, Gonen M, Fong Y, et al. Improvement in perioperative outcome after hepatic resection: analysis of 1,803 consecutive cases over the past decade. Ann Surg 2002;236:397–406 [discussion: 406–407].
50. Kooby DA, Stockman J, Ben-Porat L, et al. Influence of transfusions on perioperative and long-term outcome in patients following hepatic resection for colorectal metastases. Ann Surg 2003;237:860–9 [discussion: 869–870].
51. Milsom JW, Bohm B, Hammerhofer KA, et al. A prospective, randomized trial comparing laparoscopic versus conventional techniques in colorectal cancer surgery: a preliminary report. J Am Coll Surg 1998;187:46–54.
52. Oshikiri T, Yasuda T, Kawasaki K, et al. Hand-assisted laparoscopic surgery (HALS) is associated with less-restrictive ventilatory impairment and less risk for pulmonary complication than open laparotomy in thoracoscopic esophagectomy. Surgery 2016;159:459–66.
53. DeSouza A, Domajnko B, Park J, et al. Incisional hernia, midline versus low transverse incision: what is the ideal incision for specimen extraction and handassisted laparoscopy? Surg Endosc 2011;25:1031–6.
54. Kisielinski K, Conze J, Murken AH, et al. The Pfannenstiel or so called "bikini cut": still effective more than 100 years after first description. Hernia 2004;8:177–81.
55. Katz SC, Shia J, Liau KH, et al. Operative blood loss independently predicts recurrence and survival after resection of hepatocellular carcinoma. Ann Surg 2009;249:617–23.
56. Liu CL, Fan ST, Lo CM, et al. Anterior approach for major right hepatic resection for large hepatocellular carcinoma. Ann Surg 2000;232:25–31.
57. Hayashi N, Egami H, Kai M, et al. No-touch isolation technique reduces intraoperative shedding of tumor cells into the portal vein during resection of colorectal cancer. Surgery 1999;125:369–74.
58. Cipriani F, Fantini C, Ratti F, et al. Laparoscopic liver resections for hepatocellular carcinoma. Can we extend the surgical indication in cirrhotic patients? Surg Endosc 2018;32:617.
59. Taura K, Ikai I, Hatano E, et al. Influence of coexisting cirrhosis on outcomes after partial hepatic resection for hepato- cellular carcinoma fulfilling the Milan criteria: an analysis of 293 patients. Surgery 2007;142:685–94.
60. Poon RT, Fan ST, Ng IO, et al. Dif- ferent risk factors and prognosis for early and late intrahepatic recurrence after resection of hepatocellular carcinoma. Cancer 2000;89:500–7.
61. Farges O, Malassagne B, Flejou JF, et al. Risk of major liver re- section in patients with underlying chronic liver disease: a reappraisal. Ann Surg 1999;229:210–5.

62. Kanazawa A, Tsukamoto T, Shimizu S, et al. Impact of laparoscopic liver resection for hepatocellular carcinoma with F4-liver cirrhosis. Surg Endosc 2013;27: 2592–7.
63. Chirica M, Scatton O, Massault PP, et al. Treatment of stage IVA hepatocellular carcinoma. Should we reappraise the role of surgery? Arch Surg 2008;143: 538–43.
64. Belghiti J, Hiramatsu K, Benoist S, et al. Seven hundred forty-seven hep- atectomies in the 1990 s: an update to evaluate the actual risk of liver resection. J Am Coll Surg 2000;191:38–46.
65. Fan ST. Problems of hepatectomy in cirrhosis. Hepatogastroenterology 1998; 45(Suppl 3):1288–90.
66. Vauthey JN, Dixon E, Abdalla EK, et al. Pretreatment assessment of hep- atocellular carcinoma: expert consensus statement. HPB (Oxford) 2010;12:289–99.
67. Belli G, Fantini C, D'Agostino A, et al. Laparoscopic ver- sus open liver resection for hepatocellular car- cinoma in patients with histologically proven cirrhosis: short- and middle-term results. Surg Endosc 2007;21:2004–11.
68. Morise Z, Ciria R, Cherqui D, et al. Can we expand the indications for laparo- scopic liver resection? A systematic review and meta-analysis of laparoscopic liver resection for patients with hepatocellular carcinoma and chronic liver dis- ease. J Hepatobiliary Pancreat Sci 2015;22:342–52.
69. Xu H, Liu F, Li H, et al. Outcomes following laparoscopic versus open major hep- atectomy for hepatocellular carcinoma in patients with cirrhosis:a propensity score-matched analysis. Surg Endosc 2018;32:712.
70. Beard RE, Wang Y, Khan S, et al. Laparoscopic liver resection for hepatocellular carcinoma in early and advanced cirrhosis. HPB (Oxford) 2018;20(6):521–9.
71. Guro H, Cho JY, Han HS, et al. Laparoscopic liver resection of hepatocellular car- cinoma located in segments 7 or 8. Surg Endosc 2018;32:872.
72. Lai EC, Tang CN. Long-term survival analysis of robotic versus conventional lapa- roscopic hepatectomy for hepatocellular carcinoma: a comparative study. Surg Laparosc Endosc Percutan Tech 2016;26(2):162–6.
73. Tsung A, Geller DA, Sukato DC, et al. Robotic versus laparoscopic hepatectomy: a matched comparison. Ann Surg 2014;259(3):549–55.
74. Soubrane O, Goumard C, Laurent A, et al. Laparoscopic resection of hepatocel- lular carcinoma: a French survey in 351 patients. HPB (Oxford) 2014;16:357–65.
75. Laurent A, Tayar C, Andreoletti M, et al. Laparoscopic liver resection facilitates salvage liver transplantation for hepatocellular carcinoma. J Hepatobiliary Pan- creat Surg 2009;16:310–4.
76. Kazaryan AM, Pavlik Marangos I, Rosseland AR, et al. Laparoscopic liver re- sec- tion for malignant and benign lesions: ten- year Norwegian single-center experi- ence. Arch Surg 2010;145:34–40.
77. Hu M, Zhao G, Xu D, et al. Laparoscopic repeat resection of recurrent hepatocel- lular carcinoma. World J Surg 2011;35(3):648–55.
78. Shelat VG, Serin K, Samim M, et al. Outcomes of repeat laparoscopic liver resec- tion compared to the primary resection. World J Surg 2014;38(12):3175–80.
79. El-Gendi A, El-Shafei M, El-Gendi S, et al. Laparoscopic versus open hepatic resection for solitary hepatocellular carcinoma less than 5 cm in cirrhotic patients: a randomized controlled study. J Laparoendosc Adv Surg Tech A 2018;28: 302–10.

Minimally Invasive Management of Secondary Liver Cancer

Lavanya Yohanathan, MD, Sean P. Cleary, MD, MSc, MPH, FRCSC*

KEYWORDS

- Secondary liver disease • Laparoscopic liver surgery • Colorectal liver metastases

KEY POINTS

- The main secondary liver cancer currently managed minimally invasively is colorectal liver metastasis.
- Because the understanding of tumor biology of noncolorectal liver metastases increases, secondary liver cancer from noncolorectal origins, such as neuroendocrine tumors, other gastrointestinal tract malignancies, or breast, can be managed using minimally invasive techniques.
- Because secondary liver cancer is a systemic disease, the reduced morbidity of a minimally invasive approach allows an early return to systemic chemotherapy and reduces morbidity.

INTRODUCTION

The first laparoscopic liver resection (LLR) was published by Gagner and colleagues[1] in 1992 when they described the resection of a lesion that was determined to be focal nodular hyperplasia on final pathology examination. From this report, surgeons began to take an interest in minimally invasive hepatic resection, limiting themselves predominantly to lesions that were peripherally located and could be treated by nonanatomic wedge resections. As confidence and experience progressed, surgeons added left lateral segmentectomy as a common procedure; however, because of the oncologic concerns expressed in the 1990s, surgeons gained experience predominantly in procedures performed for benign disease. Primary liver cancers dominated the early literature not only in Asia but in other regions. For example, Cherqui and colleagues[2]

Disclosure: Dr L. Yohanathan has no relevant financial or nonfinancial relationships to disclose. Dr S.P. Cleary has no relevant financial relationships to disclose. Dr S.P. Cleary serves as a consultant for Ethicon and Erbe.
Mayo Clinic, Division of Surgery, Department of Hepatobiliary and Pancreas Surgery 200 First Street South West, Rochester, MN 55905, USA
* Corresponding author.
E-mail address: cleary.sean@mayo.edu

published an early case series of 30 patients in which 12 patients had resection for malignant disease, of which 2 out of 3 were for hepatocellular carcinoma (HCC).

As laparoscopic techniques developed and experience with these new approaches increased, case series reported expanded indications from benign conditions to malignant disease, including secondary liver metastases. For example, Koffron and colleagues[3] published their experience and evaluation of 300 minimally invasive liver resections in which metastatic disease accounted for 60 out of 300 cases.

Over the last 2 decades, advances in radiological imaging, surgical technique, and collaborative treatment protocols with interventional radiology have led to significant advances in minimally invasive hepatic resections. Meanwhile, the dramatic advances in systemic therapy and enhanced understanding of tumor biology have had profound impacts on the management of metastatic cancer, and liver metastases in particular. This progress has led to an increasingly aggressive approach to liver metastases associated with colorectal and neuroendocrine cancers and evolving roles in other malignancies (eg, breast cancer). This expansion of indications for liver resection has been accompanied by efforts to reduce the morbidity of hepatic surgery and increasing adoption of minimally invasive surgical approaches.

The main barriers to acceptance of laparoscopic liver surgery stemmed from the technical challenges associated with lesion localization, adequate techniques for parenchymal transection, difficulties controlling bleeding laparoscopically, and concerns of inferior oncologic outcomes.[2,4-6] In 2008, 45 experts in hepatobiliary surgery participated in a consensus conference in Louisville, Kentucky, to address the current world position on laparoscopic liver surgery.[7] The consensus conference suggested that solitary lesions may be the optimal indication for LLR, which can be disadvantageous for patients with secondary liver malignancies, who frequently have multiple lesions. Although the 2008 consensus emphasized the benefits of laparoscopic resections for small, solitary peripheral lesions less than or equal to 5 cm in size, high-volume centers began to report their experience with laparoscopic resection of liver lesions larger than 5 cm.[8-10]

Reports began to emerge that LLR can be safely done for patients with colorectal liver metastases (CRLMs) in lesions beyond the suggested size criteria in the Louisville statement. Nomi and colleagues[11] conducted a propensity-matched analysis between patients undergoing laparoscopic resection for tumors greater than or equal to 5 cm versus less than 5 cm. They concluded that tumor size did not influence short-term and long-term outcomes in CRLMs. Moreover, multivariate analysis revealed that tumor size was not a significant prognostic factor, whereas positive surgical margins and synchronous presentation were associated with inferior outcomes. Clear surgical margins (R0) were achieved in more than 90% of the patients with large CRLMs in this series. A propensity-matched analysis of appropriately matched types (major, minor) of resection validated a laparoscopic approach in patients with large CRLMs.

The gradual growth in application of laparoscopic resection for metastatic disease may be explained by the increasing technical advancements in laparoscopy, increased experience, and increased technical expertise of the operating surgeons as well as the utility of intraoperative ultrasonography to allow safe decision making with regard to lesion localization and identification of relevant biliary and vascular structures.[12] Specifically, ultrasonography is particularly important when treating metastases to the liver in order to account for all metastases, identify metastases missed on axial imaging, and guide surgical resection. A case-control study by Langella and colleagues[13] assessed the oncologic safety of ultrasonography-guided LLR for CRLM. When comparing laparoscopic versus open case-matched patients, the oncologic safety of ultrasonography-assisted LLR for CRLM was confirmed.[13]

The most recent consensus conference on the status of laparoscopic liver surgery was held in Morioka, Japan, in 2014 and provided recommendations to aid its future development. An impartial jury concluded that minor LLRs had become standard practice because of the consistency of evidence showing decreased perioperative morbidity and equivalent oncologic outcomes, whereas major liver resections were still innovative procedures in the exploration phase because there were limited data from highly specialized centers. There was general agreement that laparoscopic liver surgery had expanded in its indications and is not limited by size criteria or the number of lesions, reflecting a large body of literature on the use of the minimally invasive approach for metastatic disease to the liver.[14]

In 2009, Nguyen and colleagues[15] published a detailed review of almost 3000 cases, highlighting the most common indications, contraindications, various types of laparoscopic procedures performed, and complications based on their review of 127 original articles. Only 50% of laparoscopic liver procedures were performed for malignancy, of which 52% were for HCC and the remaining 35% were for CRLM. The investigators also highlighted a conversion-to-open rate of 4.1% with bleeding as the most common indication, whereas other common reasons for conversion were adhesions, anatomic limitations, poor exposure, proximity to major vascular structures, lack of progression, gross positive tumor margin, equipment failure, satellite lesions beyond planned resection, requirement of associated surgical procedure, and large tumor size. The investigators concluded that, in experienced hands, LLRs are safe, with acceptable morbidity and mortality for both minor and major hepatic resections. From an oncologic standpoint, the 3-year and 5-year survival rates for both HCC and CRLM were comparable with open surgery.

In 2016, Ciria and colleagues[16] published a meta-analysis on LLRs of 9527 patients. Here, 65% of diagnoses were for malignant disease and 35% were for benign conditions, indicating that, over a 7-year period since the Nguyen and colleagues[15] publication, there was a 15% increase in the relative proportion laparoscopic liver surgery for malignant disease. When matching 2900 cases between laparoscopic and open arms, there was no increased mortality and significantly less complications, transfusions, blood loss, and hospital stay favoring the laparoscopic arm. It is important to highlight that geographic variation has a strong impact on surgical indications when looking at the published literature and its impact on trends of uptake throughout the world. Most of the Eastern literature is focused on resection for HCC as opposed to the Western series in which CRLM is the leading diagnosis. Comparison of these two publications shows the evolution of the field over that time, with improving safety and perioperative outcomes in LLR.

LAPAROSCOPIC SURGERY FOR COLORECTAL LIVER METASTASES

CRLMs occur in 40% to 50% of all patients diagnosed with colorectal cancer, of which 15% to 25% are synchronous and the remaining 25% to 40% develop metastases after resection of the primary colonic malignancy (metachronous presentation).[17–19] Although 5-year survival rates following curative liver resection range from 35% to 58%, two-thirds of these patients develop tumor recurrence, and 40% of these recurrences are limited to the liver.[17,20–22] Although there have been significant improvements in the management of stage IV colorectal cancer over the past few decades, surgical resection of the primary and metastatic lesions in combination with systemic chemotherapy offers the only chance for long-term survival.

With the advent and expansion of indications and use of laparoscopic liver surgery, this approach has been favorable in simultaneous resection as well as the liver-first approach.[23] Many studies have shown that there are benefits of the minimally invasive approach on short-term outcomes as well as long-term outcomes without compromising oncologic results.[24] To summarize, as indications for minimally invasive liver surgery for colorectal metastases continue to grow, consideration of this approach on a case-by-case basis may allow quicker recovery so patients can move on to their next treatment regimens.

Impact of Laparoscopic Liver Resection on Adjuvant Chemotherapy

Three studies have shown the impact of laparoscopic liver surgery on return to adjuvant chemotherapy. They showed that the time to commencement of adjuvant therapy start was significantly shorter after LLR compared with open liver resection (OLR). Mbah and colleagues[25] investigated patients undergoing major liver resections, 40% of whom had metastatic disease from noncolorectal sites. Because baseline patient and tumor characteristics were not matched between both groups, they were not comparable between laparoscopic and open approaches. The investigators compared 44 laparoscopic cases to 76 open cases in which the extent of resection was similar. They showed that the laparoscopic group had lower blood loss (276 mL) than patients with open resection (614 mL) and had a shorter length of hospital stay (5 days) than patients with open resection (9 days). Patients with LLR had a shorter time to adjuvant chemotherapy initiation (24 days vs 39 days). Overall complication rates were higher but statistically insignificant in patients with open resection.

Tohme and colleagues[26] matched patients on a 1:1 on baseline and intraoperative variables but not on pathologic features. The analysis of time to adjuvant chemotherapy was based on expected differences in rates of complications between the laparoscopic and open groups. Shorter length of hospitalization, fewer major complications, and shorter interval to postoperative chemotherapy (median 42 vs 63 days; $P<.001$) were found in the laparoscopic arm. Unique to this study, a multivariable analysis was performed, which showed that the surgical approach was associated with timing to chemotherapy and that postoperative complications resulted in a delay to chemotherapy in those who underwent open resection. Such delays resulted in worse disease-free survival (DFS) among patients who received postoperative chemotherapy more than 60 days after surgery (67% of patients in the minimally invasive group received postoperative chemotherapy within 60 days, as opposed to 35% of patients in the open group.)

In contrast, Kawai and colleagues[27] showed a significantly shorter time to adjuvant therapy following LLR compared with an open approach using a propensity-matched analysis. They matched groups based on baseline, oncologic, and intraoperative characteristics to reach their conclusions and accounted for confounding factors. Comparing the time interval between liver resection and adjuvant chemotherapy, the start was significantly shorter in the LLR than in the OLR group (43 $\pm$ 10 days vs 55 $\pm$ 18 days; $P = .012$). Although only 34% of open patients received adjuvant chemotherapy within 8 weeks of surgery, all patients in the laparoscopic group received chemotherapy within 8 weeks.

Literature Review

Laparoscopic versus open resection for colorectal liver metastases

There have been several single and multi-institutional case series and meta-analyses comparing LLRs with OLRs.[28–40]

Castaing and colleagues[33] compared laparoscopic and open hepatectomy for CRLM among 2 specialized centers. They assessed 2 groups of patients, composed of 60 patients in each group based on an intention-to-treat analysis. The comparable cohorts consisted of 215 patients in the laparoscopic group and 1783 in the open group. The median follow-up for the laparoscopic and open group were 30 months and 33 months, respectively ($P = .75$). In comparing overall survival (OS), 1-year, 3-year, and 5-year patient survival for the laparoscopic group was 97%, 82%, and 64% ($P = .32$) compared with 97%, 70%, and 56% in the open group ($P = .32$), respectively. Similarly, DFS at 1, 3, and 5 years was 70%, 47%, and 35%, and 70%, 40%, and 27% ($P = .32$) respectively for the two groups. These data confirmed that LLR versus OLR had comparable oncologic outcomes.

Similar outcomes were shown in North America by Cannon and colleagues,[35] who compared 35 patients in the laparoscopic arm with 140 patients in the open cohort. Similar proportions of patients underwent a synchronous operation and major hepatectomy. Blood loss, complications, and duration of stay were reduced in the laparoscopic cohort. Similar rates of 5-year OS and DFS were observed in the laparoscopic and open groups (OS 36% vs 42%, $P = .818$; DFS 15% vs 22%, $P = .346$), respectively.

Zhou and colleagues[41] highlighted the merits of LLR and its advantages over open surgery in a meta-analysis of 8 retrospective studies, including the 2 previously discussed.[33,35] The meta-analyses included 695 patients and showed that laparoscopic resection was associated with significant reduction in intraoperative blood loss, need for postoperative transfusions, morbidity, and length of hospital stay. In addition, they also reported that postoperative recurrence, 5-year OS, and DFS were comparable between both groups.

A recent updated review by Berardi and colleagues[42] analyzing 2238 patients across 4 centers showed that there has been an increase in laparoscopic surgery from 5% to 43% between 2000 and 2015. Wedge resections accounted for most of the operations. With respect to outcomes, blood loss, operative time, and conversion rate significantly improved with time, with the highest percentage being in 2015. The 5-year OS rate for CRLM was 54% and the recurrence-free survival rate was 37%.

Nevertheless, the literature on patients undergoing LLR seems to suggest that they are a selected cohort consisting of patients. As the number of retrospective single-center series of LLR for CRLM grew, there was widespread acknowledgment of the aforementioned biases inherent in these reports. As a result, there was a concerted emphasis by interested surgeons to generate outcomes data from randomized controlled prospective trials that would evaluate LLR with minimal experimenter bias.

The first multicenter double-blind trial, randomized clinical trial of open versus laparoscopic left lateral hepatic sectionectomy within an enhanced recovery after surgery programme (ORANGE II) study,[43] compared laparoscopic left lateral sectionectomy with the open technique. Although the trial showed that the laparoscopic approach was associated with shorter hospital stay and reduced overall morbidity, this trial was terminated prematurely because of failure of accrual.

In addition, the first single-center, prospective superiority, randomized trial comparing laparoscopic resection versus OLR for CRLM was published in March 2017.[44] The Oslo laparoscopic versus open liver resection for colorectal metastases (Oslo-CoMet) study group assessed a total of 280 patients with resectable liver metastases who were randomly assigned to laparoscopic or open parenchymal-sparing liver resection. The primary outcome of this trial was postoperative complications within 30 days. Secondary outcomes were postoperative length of stay, blood loss, operation time, resection margins, and cost-effectiveness. When assessing primary outcomes, the postoperative complications were graded by a blind assessor and documented by nurses. The records did not indicate operative technique and described the postoperative state of the patient in 3 daily reports. Telephone interviews conducted at 1, 8, and 28 days after surgery were also documented and reviewed when collecting the data for 30-day complications.

The investigators report a postoperative complication rate of 19% in the laparoscopic group compared with 31% in the open surgery group, accounting for a 12% difference (confidence interval, 1.67–21.8; P = .021). This finding mirrored many retrospective, single-institution studies showing that postoperative morbidity was superior in the laparoscopic group. In their assessment of morbidity, the investigators excluded Accordion grade 1 complications; this analysis likely resulted in a lower absolute complication rate compared with other series but allowed a realistic comparison of clinically significant adverse outcomes. The analysis of secondary outcomes showed that the length of stay was shorter in the laparoscopic arm, and there was no difference in blood loss, operation time, and resection margins. There was no significant difference in overall 90-day mortality, with no deaths in either arm. In addition, costs were equal at the 4-month follow-up, and the investigators were able to point out that those in the laparoscopic arm had improved quality-adjusted life compared with OLR. The trial may have been subject to some bias because, although the outcomes assessor was blinded to the treatment arms, the operating surgeon was not. It must be acknowledged that this was an expert surgeon single-center trial with 400 LLRs performed before the start of this trial; hence, the applicability of the results to centers with lower volume and/or experience may be limited. In addition to this, the positive findings of this trial were limited to parenchyma-sparing liver resections, therefore consideration should be given to this particular point when using these results when undertaking laparoscopic major hepatectomies. When interpreting the results of the study, it must be pointed out that, when the investigators reported the morbidity between both groups, the margin of statistical significance was narrow.

Despite some limitations, the Oslo-CoMet trial provides an important contribution and can be considered a landmark study at this time. Although many retrospective studies suggested oncologic safety, this trial provides a prospective comparison in OS and recurrence-free survival that seems to support equivalent outcomes between laparoscopic and open approaches. Similarly, although costs have been assessed in several articles, this trial shows in a prospective fashion that the increased equipment and instrument costs with laparoscopic surgery are offset by efficiencies and savings in postoperative care. Furthermore, this study was able to extend the postoperative outcome and cost assessments beyond the primary hospital stay to referring institutions. The investigators also provide important validation to long-held beliefs of improved quality of life for patients undergoing minimally invasive liver surgery.

In summary, the literature to date shows LLRs are superior to open resection with respect to morbidity and some intraoperative parameters such as blood loss. Although the laparoscopic equipment and maintenance of a minimally invasive program are costly, the costs become equal when considering length of stay and management of postoperative morbidity. In addition, quality of life was calculated at baseline, 1 month, and 4 months via standard surveys, and patients in the laparoscopic arm had improved quality of life. Ultimately, the data from the Oslo-CoMet supported the findings of previous institutional series and retrospective reviews in that there was decreased length of stay and overall morbidity, and (importantly) equivalent oncologic outcomes.

Laparoscopic liver surgery after laparoscopic or open colorectal surgery

Di Fabio and colleagues[40] conducted a multicenter observational study of the outcomes of laparoscopic hepatectomy for colorectal metastases after open versus laparoscopic colorectal surgery. A total of 394 patients were analyzed, of whom 306 patients (78%) had prior open and 88 (22%) had prior laparoscopic colorectal resection. Of these patients, laparoscopic major hepatectomies were undertaken in 63 patients (16%). The incidence of unfavorable intraoperative incidents during laparoscopic liver surgery was significantly higher among patients who had previous open colorectal surgery (26%) compared with previous laparoscopic surgery (14%, $P = .017$).[40] The approach for primary colorectal cancer did not influence the rate of positive resection margins or postoperative complications.

The same investigators also conducted a multicenter propensity score–based analysis of short-term and long-term outcomes to justify the use of LLR for colorectal metastases in elderly and octogenarian patients. A total of 775 patients were included and, after propensity matching, 225 patients were comparable in each of the main groups (the cohort was divided into 3 subgroups based on age). There was less blood loss, less overall morbidity, and shorter high dependency unit and total hospital stays in the laparoscopic group. However, there was a gradual loss of these advantages with increasing age, with no statistically significant benefits in octogenarians except for a lower high dependency unit stay.[40]

Role of Laparoscopic Reresection of Colorectal Liver Metastases

As significant progress has been made in treatment of CRLM, with up to 60% 5-year survival rates, an increasingly common occurrence is rerecurrence of cancer. Management of rerecurrent colorectal metastases after prior surgical resection is increasingly recognized, often leading to consideration of reresection. Repeat liver resection is fraught with complications related to technical challenges.

Repeat resection of CRLM is indicated in these patients in our opinion, provided they are technically resectable with preservation of future liver remnant volume. This point is discussed as a multidisciplinary approach for appropriate sequencing of treatment between chemotherapy and timing of repeat resection.

Shafaee and colleagues[45] described the first large series among 3 institutions with respect to repeat LLRs. Most of the patients that they analyzed were for metastatic disease (63 patients), and the remainder were for HCC and benign tumors (13 patients). All of the patients in the cohort had undergone previous liver resection, and 58% of patients had previous laparoscopic resection, as opposed to 37% who had open procedures, including 16 major resections (en bloc removal of 3 or more Couinaud segments). Of these patients, 11% required conversion to an open procedure. Reasons for conversion were adhesions, excessive intraoperative bleeding, and failure to progress caused by tumor location. Most patients (64%) had wedge resections, whereas 25% of patients had major hepatectomies.

Patients who had previous open procedures had greater intraoperative blood loss and transfusion requirements compared with the previous laparoscopic group. There was no significant difference between postoperative complications and duration of hospital stay between patients. The 3-year and 5-year actuarial survival rates were 83% and 55% between the laparoscopic and open groups respectively. Based on this, the investigators concluded that a laparoscopic approach is a safe alternative to open surgery specifically in patients who had previous laparoscopic resections.[45]

When analyzing such a study, selection bias and the differences between tumor and patient characteristics between the 2 groups are important issues to keep in mind. To this end, there were no significant differences with respect to demographic parameters and type of procedure performed. Other investigators have supported this view, adding that repeat LLRs are safe, feasible, and can be performed with minimal morbidity; however, it is technically challenging compared with initial laparoscopic resection.[46] The largest analysis of patients was performed with a multicenter propensity-matched analysis with respect to short-term and long-term outcomes.[47] Here again, there was evidence to support consideration of laparoscopic repeat hepatectomy; however, considering that outcomes were different among both groups, emphasis on patient selection is of utmost importance.

Technical Considerations

It is of utmost importance to review factors associated with morbidity following surgical resection. Patients treated with neoadjuvant chemotherapy have specific considerations with respect to chemotherapy-induced liver toxicity. This consideration in turn affects the safety of the liver resection, and, specifically with soft livers, this should be anticipated and addressed when using a laparoscopic approach (**Table 1**).

Table 1 Technical considerations and pearls of laparoscopic liver surgery	
1	Chemotherapy affects the consistency and quality of the liver during liver resection. The liver may be difficult to manipulate because of friability and increased bleeding A laparoscopic approach has been shown to reduce the effects of bleeding caused by pneumoperitoneum and has advantages in these patients. Gentle tissue handling must be encouraged during these procedures
2	Prevention of bleeding and anatomic considerations are enhanced by the use of intraoperative ultrasonography, and laparoscopic hepatobiliary surgeons must be experts in the use and interpretation of intraoperative ultrasonography
3	Paying attention to the technical limitations of laparoscopic liver surgery allows surgeons to plan appropriate trocar placement and appropriate use of instruments. Key considerations are the lack of angulation and mobilization of instruments rather than appropriate tissue handling to obtain appropriate angles and approaches
3	Metastatic disease affecting the liver is often multifocal and bilobar. To accurately treat disease, regular use and familiarity with intraoperative ultrasonography is crucial. Adjunctive therapies such as laparoscopic radiofrequency ablation may be required in combination with resection and must be arranged in appropriate cases
4	Previous surgery can pose risk of adhesions and difficulty; however, these operations can be addressed laparoscopically. Appropriate planning of trocar placement and gaining entry into the abdomen in such cases with optical trocars and Veress needle technique should be considered
5	LLR is a safe alternative and may have improved benefit in patients who are elderly or cirrhotic
6	Repeat laparoscopic hepatectomy is safe and technically feasible but may be fraught with complications. The liver parenchyma is friable, and these patients usually have added changes secondary to preoperative chemotherapy. Consideration to future liver remnant and appropriate precautions must be taken (ie, ALPPS, portal vein embolization)
7	Be cautious of changes in the portal dissection and altered anatomy following portal vein embolization. Familiarity with laparoscopic inflow occlusion is essential when performing laparoscopic hepatectomy, particularly after portal vein embolization and repeat resections
8	Parenchymal preservation is associated with decreased morbidity and does not compromise oncologic outcomes[48,49]
9	Laparoscopic liver surgery allows patients a shorter recovery time and hence quicker receipt of adjuvant chemotherapy, whether definitive or a bridge for subsequent surgery

Abbreviation: ALPPS, associating liver partition and portal vein ligation for staged hepatectomy.

LAPAROSCOPIC SURGERY FOR OTHER SECONDARY DISEASES TO THE LIVER

Although most LLRs for secondary malignancy of the liver are related to CRLM, a substantial number of patients undergo LLR for non-CRLM indications.

Neuroendocrine Liver Metastases

Neuroendocrine tumors are considered to have an indolent and chronic course. The accepted 5-year survival rate for all types of carcinoid tumors is 67.2%.[50] The presence of liver metastases is associated with worse survival regardless of the primary site of disease. These tumors generally have a 5-year survival of 75% to 99%, but only 20% of patients survive greater than 5 years when they present with unresectable liver metastases.[51–53] Carcinoid liver metastases are fairly indolent and potentially require multiple interventions over time. A laparoscopic approach may offer advantages for this disease entity because repeat operations on the liver may be warranted when recurrences do occur.

Kandil and colleagues[54] conducted the first comparative institutional series on laparoscopic versus open resection of neuroendocrine metastases. The laparoscopic group had less mean operative time, less blood loss, and a shorter hospital stay (P<.05 for all). Complications were similar in both groups and the 3-year DFS for the laparoscopic group was 73.3% compared with 47.6% for the open group. The investigators do highlight that there was a considerable amount of selection bias and that LLR was chosen for patients with 4 or fewer metastases. Patients with advanced tumors or those in more challenging locations were treated with open surgery. In addition, some of these cases were hand assisted earlier in their experience.

In summary, a laparoscopic approach may be considered in patients who have limited liver metastases. Patients who have the need for associated bowel resection with mesenteric lymphadenectomies may be better served with an open approach.

Breast Cancer

The role of metastasectomy for breast cancer metastases to the liver has been reported in systematic reviews and several institutional series. A recently published systematic review included patients with breast cancer who underwent hepatic resection in the absence of other extrahepatic disease. Median survival rates ranged from 29.5 to 116 months. In patients presenting with oligometastatic disease, 5-year survival rates ranged from 21% to 57%, with median survival ranging from 32 to 58 months. These analyses justify consideration for resection in patients with breast cancer liver metastases. Consideration should be given to presence of isolated or multiple metastases because the investigators did notice that there was an increase in 30-day morbidity (14%–42%).[55]

Some investigators have extrapolated results from resection of colorectal metastases to guide their management principles for metastases from other primaries, including patients with limited comorbidities, 4 or fewer liver tumors, and no (or limited and stable) extrahepatic disease on preoperative imaging. Laparoscopic radiofrequency ablation was an option in patients with prohibitive surgical risk, with 4 or fewer liver tumors all less than 4 cm in size, tumors located more than 1 cm from the central biliary structures, and no (or limited and stable) extrahepatic disease on preoperative imaging. Hormone receptor and human epidermal growth factor receptor 2 status was not a determining factor for patient selection. Preoperative chemotherapy was used at the discretion of the referring oncologist or surgeon.[56]

There have been several case reports for the role of hepatic metastasectomy in other secondary diseases, including gastric,[57,58] breast,[59] and gynecologic cancers,[60] for the role of debulking, and in renal cell cancer.[61] Consideration should be given to the extent of operation, DFS, patterns of recurrence, and goals of surgery. All of these factors must be considered when considering a laparoscopic approach. The most important considerations are the biology of each tumor and prognostic factors related to the primary tumor when considering the role of resection of liver metastases.

Other

Both ovarian and germ cell tumors are chemosensitive; however, recent data and current trials are designed to emphasize the importance of debulking surgery in these patients, including those leading to liver metastases.[62] These patients, similar to those who undergo repeat surgery for CRLM, should be considered for laparoscopic resection. Often, the location of these lesions is not deep within the parenchyma, making a laparoscopic approach feasible.

An appropriate management plan, including the decision to perform a minimally invasive resection for metastases not of colorectal, neuroendocrine, or ovarian origin, has to be tailored to the individual patient.[63]

SUMMARY

At the current time, there is an important role for laparoscopic liver surgery for secondary liver cancer. Innovation and change based on an understanding gained from open surgery has allowed progress in the surgical treatment of these patients. With further and more widespread adoption of laparoscopy, indications will continue to expand and increasingly complex procedures will be performed.

REFERENCES

1. Gagner M, Lacroix A, Prinz RA, et al. Early experience with laparoscopic approach for adrenalectomy. Surgery 1993;114(6):1120–4 [discussion: 24–5].
2. Cherqui D, Husson E, Hammoud R, et al. Laparoscopic liver resections: a feasibility study in 30 patients. Ann Surg 2000;232(6):753–62.
3. Koffron AJ, Auffenberg G, Kung R, et al. Evaluation of 300 minimally invasive liver resections at a single institution: less is more. Ann Surg 2007;246(3):385–92 [discussion: 92–4].
4. Cherqui D. Laparoscopic liver resection. Br J Surg 2003;90(6):644–6.
5. D'Albuquerque LA, Herman P. Laparoscopic hepatectomy: is it a reality? Arq Gastroenterol 2006;43(3):243–6 [in Portuguese].
6. Vigano L, Tayar C, Laurent A, et al. Laparoscopic liver resection: a systematic review. J Hepatobiliary Pancreat Surg 2009;16(4):410–21.
7. Buell JF, Cherqui D, Geller DA, et al. The international position on laparoscopic liver surgery: the Louisville statement, 2008. Ann Surg 2009;250(5):825–30.
8. Ai JH, Li JW, Chen J, et al. Feasibility and safety of laparoscopic liver resection for hepatocellular carcinoma with a tumor size of 5-10 cm. PLoS One 2013;8(8): e72328.
9. Doughtie CA, Egger ME, Cannon RM, et al. Laparoscopic hepatectomy is a safe and effective approach for resecting large colorectal liver metastases. Am Surg 2013;79(6):566–71.
10. Shelat VG, Cipriani F, Basseres T, et al. Pure laparoscopic liver resection for large malignant tumors: does size matter? Ann Surg Oncol 2015;22(4):1288–93.

11. Nomi T, Fuks D, Louvet C, et al. Outcomes of laparoscopic liver resection for patients with large colorectal liver metastases: a case-matched analysis. World J Surg 2016;40(7):1702–8.

12. Ellebaek SB, Fristrup CW, Mortensen MB. Laparoscopic ultrasound imaging in colorectal cancer resection may increase the detection rate of small liver metastases. Ugeskr Laeger 2016;178(24) [pii:V01160007] [in Danish].

13. Langella S, Russolillo N, D'Eletto M, et al. Oncological safety of ultrasound-guided laparoscopic liver resection for colorectal metastases: a case-control study. Updates Surg 2015;67(2):147–55.

14. Wakabayashi G, Cherqui D, Geller DA, et al. Recommendations for laparoscopic liver resection: a report from the second international consensus conference held in Morioka. Ann Surg 2015;261(4):619–29.

15. Nguyen KT, Gamblin TC, Geller DA. World review of laparoscopic liver resection—2,804 patients. Ann Surg 2009;250(5):831–41.

16. Ciria R, Cherqui D, Geller DA, et al. Comparative short-term benefits of laparoscopic liver resection: 9000 cases and climbing. Ann Surg 2016;263(4):761–77.

17. Hughes KS, Simon R, Songhorabodi S, et al. Resection of the liver for colorectal carcinoma metastases: a multi-institutional study of patterns of recurrence. Surgery 1986;100(2):278–84.

18. Nordlinger B, Sorbye H, Glimelius B, et al. Perioperative FOLFOX4 chemotherapy and surgery versus surgery alone for resectable liver metastases from colorectal cancer (EORTC 40983): long-term results of a randomised, controlled, phase 3 trial. Lancet Oncol 2013;14(12):1208–15.

19. Nordlinger B, Sorbye H, Glimelius B, et al. Perioperative chemotherapy with FOLFOX4 and surgery versus surgery alone for resectable liver metastases from colorectal cancer (EORTC Intergroup trial 40983): a randomised controlled trial. Lancet 2008;371(9617):1007–16.

20. Fong Y, Fortner J, Sun RL, et al. Clinical score for predicting recurrence after hepatic resection for metastatic colorectal cancer: analysis of 1001 consecutive cases. Ann Surg 1999;230(3):309–18 [discussion: 18–21].

21. Sharma S, Camci C, Jabbour N. Management of hepatic metastasis from colorectal cancers: an update. J Hepatobiliary Pancreat Surg 2008;15(6):570–80.

22. Jamison RL, Donohue JH, Nagorney DM, et al. Hepatic resection for metastatic colorectal cancer results in cure for some patients. Arch Surg 1997;132(5): 505–10 [discussion: 11].

23. Gorgun E, Yazici P, Onder A, et al. Laparoscopic versus open 1-stage resection of synchronous liver metastases and primary colorectal cancer. Gland Surg 2017; 6(4):324–9.

24. Garritano S, Selvaggi F, Spampinato MG. Simultaneous minimally invasive treatment of colorectal neoplasm with synchronous liver metastasis. Biomed Res Int 2016;2016:9328250.

25. Mbah N, Agle SC, Philips P, et al. Laparoscopic hepatectomy significantly shortens the time to postoperative chemotherapy in patients undergoing major hepatectomies. Am J Surg 2017;213(6):1060–4.

26. Tohme S, Goswami J, Han K, et al. Minimally invasive resection of colorectal cancer liver metastases leads to an earlier initiation of chemotherapy compared to open surgery. J Gastrointest Surg 2015;19(12):2199–206.

27. Kawai T, Goumard C, Jeune F, et al. Laparoscopic liver resection for colorectal liver metastasis patients allows patients to start adjuvant chemotherapy without delay: a propensity score analysis. Surg Endosc 2018. https://doi.org/10.1007/s00464-018-6046-y.

28. Gigot JF, Glineur D, Santiago Azagra J, et al. Laparoscopic liver resection for malignant liver tumors: preliminary results of a multicenter European study. Ann Surg 2002;236(1):90–7.

29. O'Rourke N, Shaw I, Nathanson L, et al. Laparoscopic resection of hepatic colorectal metastases. HPB (Oxford) 2004;6(4):230–5.

30. Vibert E, Perniceni T, Levard H, et al. Laparoscopic liver resection. Br J Surg 2006;93(1):67–72.

31. Tang CN, Tsui KK, Ha JP, et al. A single-centre experience of 40 laparoscopic liver resections. Hong Kong Med J 2006;12(6):419–25.

32. Mala T, Edwin B, Gladhaug I, et al. A comparative study of the short-term outcome following open and laparoscopic liver resection of colorectal metastases. Surg Endosc 2002;16(7):1059–63.

33. Castaing D, Vibert E, Ricca L, et al. Oncologic results of laparoscopic versus open hepatectomy for colorectal liver metastases in two specialized centers. Ann Surg 2009;250(5):849–55.

34. Abu Hilal M, Underwood T, Zuccaro M, et al. Short- and medium-term results of totally laparoscopic resection for colorectal liver metastases. Br J Surg 2010; 97(6):927–33.

35. Cannon RM, Scoggins CR, Callender GG, et al. Laparoscopic versus open resection of hepatic colorectal metastases. Surgery 2012;152(4):567–73 [discussion: 73–4].

36. Cheung TT, Poon RT, Yuen WK, et al. Outcome of laparoscopic versus open hepatectomy for colorectal liver metastases. ANZ J Surg 2013;83(11):847–52.

37. Topal H, Tiek J, Aerts R, et al. Outcome of laparoscopic major liver resection for colorectal metastases. Surg Endosc 2012;26(9):2451–5.

38. Guerron AD, Aliyev S, Agcaoglu O, et al. Laparoscopic versus open resection of colorectal liver metastasis. Surg Endosc 2013;27(4):1138–43.

39. Qiu J, Chen S, Pankaj P, et al. Laparoscopic hepatectomy for hepatic colorectal metastases – a retrospective comparative cohort analysis and literature review. PLoS One 2013;8(3):e60153.

40. Di Fabio F, Barkhatov L, Bonadio I, et al. The impact of laparoscopic versus open colorectal cancer surgery on subsequent laparoscopic resection of liver metastases: a multicenter study. Surgery 2015;157(6):1046–54.

41. Zhou Y, Xiao Y, Wu L, et al. Laparoscopic liver resection as a safe and efficacious alternative to open resection for colorectal liver metastasis: a meta-analysis. BMC Surg 2013;13:44.

42. Berardi G, Van Cleven S, Fretland AA, et al. Evolution of laparoscopic liver surgery from innovation to implementation to mastery: perioperative and oncologic outcomes of 2,238 patients from 4 European specialized centers. J Am Coll Surg 2017;225(5):639–49.

43. Wong-Lun-Hing EM, van Dam RM, van Breukelen GJ, et al. Randomized clinical trial of open versus laparoscopic left lateral hepatic sectionectomy within an enhanced recovery after surgery programme (ORANGE II study). Br J Surg 2017;104(5):525–35.

44. Fretland AA, Dagenborg VJ, Bjornelv GMW, et al. Laparoscopic versus open resection for colorectal liver metastases: the OSLO-COMET randomized controlled trial. Ann Surg 2018;267(2):199–207.

45. Shafaee Z, Kazaryan AM, Marvin MR, et al. Is laparoscopic repeat hepatectomy feasible? A tri-institutional analysis. J Am Coll Surg 2011;212(2):171–9.

46. Shelat VG, Serin K, Samim M, et al. Outcomes of repeat laparoscopic liver resection compared to the primary resection. World J Surg 2014;38(12):3175–80.

47. Hallet J, Sa Cunha A, Cherqui D, et al. Laparoscopic compared to open repeat hepatectomy for colorectal liver metastases: a multi-institutional propensity-matched analysis of short- and long-term outcomes. World J Surg 2017;41(12): 3189–98.

48. Gold JS, Are C, Kornprat P, et al. Increased use of parenchymal-sparing surgery for bilateral liver metastases from colorectal cancer is associated with improved mortality without change in oncologic outcome: trends in treatment over time in 440 patients. Ann Surg 2008;247(1):109–17.

49. Kingham TP, Correa-Gallego C, D'Angelica MI, et al. Hepatic parenchymal preservation surgery: decreasing morbidity and mortality rates in 4,152 resections for malignancy. J Am Coll Surg 2015;220(4):471–9.

50. Modlin IM, Lye KD, Kidd M. A 5-decade analysis of 13,715 carcinoid tumors. Cancer 2003;97(4):934–59.

51. Rindi G, D'Adda T, Froio E, et al. Prognostic factors in gastrointestinal endocrine tumors. Endocr Pathol 2007;18(3):145–9.

52. Frilling A, Sotiropoulos GC, Li J, et al. Multimodal management of neuroendocrine liver metastases. HPB (Oxford) 2010;12(6):361–79.

53. Mayo SC, de Jong MC, Bloomston M, et al. Surgery versus intra-arterial therapy for neuroendocrine liver metastasis: a multicenter international analysis. Ann Surg Oncol 2011;18(13):3657–65.

54. Kandil E, Noureldine SI, Koffron A, et al. Outcomes of laparoscopic and open resection for neuroendocrine liver metastases. Surgery 2012;152(6):1225–31.

55. Tasleem S, Bolger JC, Kelly ME, et al. The role of liver resection in patients with metastatic breast cancer: a systematic review examining the survival impact. Ir J Med Sci 2018. https://doi.org/10.1007/s11845-018-1746-9.

56. Cassera MA, Hammill CW, Ujiki MB, et al. Surgical management of breast cancer liver metastases. HPB (Oxford) 2011;13(4):272–8.

57. Morise Z, Sugioka A, Hoshimoto S, et al. The role of hepatectomy for patients with liver metastases of gastric cancer. Hepatogastroenterology 2008;55(85): 1238–41.

58. Makino H, Kunisaki C, Izumisawa Y, et al. Indication for hepatic resection in the treatment of liver metastasis from gastric cancer. Anticancer Res 2010;30(6): 2367–76.

59. van Walsum GA, de Ridder JA, Verhoef C, et al. Resection of liver metastases in patients with breast cancer: survival and prognostic factors. Eur J Surg Oncol 2012;38(10):910–7.

60. Bosquet JG, Merideth MA, Podratz KC, et al. Hepatic resection for metachronous metastases from ovarian carcinoma. HPB (Oxford) 2006;8(2):93–6.

61. Langan RC, Ripley RT, Davis JL, et al. Liver directed therapy for renal cell carcinoma. J Cancer 2012;3:184–90.

62. Li J, Wu X. Current strategy for the treatment of ovarian germ cell tumors: role of extensive surgery. Curr Treat Options Oncol 2016;17(8):44.

63. Labgaa I, Slankamenac K, Schadde E, et al. Liver resection for metastases not of colorectal, neuroendocrine, sarcomatous, or ovarian (NCNSO) origin: a multicentric study. Am J Surg 2018;215(1):125–30.

Minimally Invasive Surgery for Gallbladder Cancer

Eduardo A. Vega, MD[a,b,1], Marcel Sanhueza, MD[c,2], Eduardo Viñuela, MD[c,d],*

KEYWORDS

- Gallbladder neoplasms • Minimally invasive surgery • Laparoscopy
- Surgical technique

KEY POINTS

- Extended oncologic resection is recommended for patients with incidental and nonincidental gallbladder cancer in whom no contraindication exists.
- The extended resection can be completed safely with a minimally invasive approach with reduction in morbidity.
- High-quality data comparing oncologic outcomes between open and minimally invasive approach are lacking, but preliminary data suggest that a minimally invasive approach is safe.
- A systematic approach with predefined steps helps in adopting and executing the minimally invasive approach.
- In general, technical steps must include cystic stump resection (if safely feasible), liver resection, and lymph node dissection.

 Video content accompanies this article at http://www.surgonc.theclinics.com.

INTRODUCTION

Although gallbladder cancer (GBC) is considered to be relatively rare in the United States, with an incidence of 1.1 per 100,000, it is the most common malignancy of

---

Disclosure: None of the authors have conflicts of interest.
[a] Department of Surgical Oncology, The University of Texas MD Anderson Cancer Center, 1400 Hermann Pressler FCT17.5065, Unit 1484, Houston, Texas, USA; [b] Department of Surgery, Hepato-bilio-pancreatic Surgery Unit, Hospital Sotero Del Rio, Concha y Toro Avenue 3459, Puente Alto, Santiago 8207257, Chile; [c] Department of Digestive Surgery, Faculty of Medicine, Catholic University of Chile, Avenida Libertador Bernardo O'Higgins 390, Santiago 8331150, Chile; [d] Department of Digestive Surgery, Faculty Medicine, Catholic University of Chile, Sotero del Rio Hospital, Concha y Toro Avenue 3459, Puente Alto, Santiago 8207257, Chile
[1] Present address: 1400 Hermann Pressler FCT17.5065, Unit 1484, Houston, Texas 77030-4009, USA.
[2] Present address: Avendia Libertador Bernardo O'Higgins 340, Santiago, Región Metropolitana, Chile.
* Corresponding author. Department of Digestive Surgery, Faculty Medicine, Catholic University of Chile, Sotero del Rio Hospital, Concha y Toro Avenue 3459, Puente Alto, Chile.
E-mail address: evinuela@uc.cl

Surg Oncol Clin N Am 28 (2019) 243–253
https://doi.org/10.1016/j.soc.2018.11.001
1055-3207/19/© 2018 Elsevier Inc. All rights reserved.

the biliary system, accounting for 80% to 95% of biliary tract cancers.[1,2] GBC is a highly aggressive cancer and is associated with a poor prognosis: the 5-year survival rate is less than 10% for those who present with disease at an advanced stage, accounting for 3800 deaths annually.[3]

There is marked geographic variation in the incidence and mortality of GBC, both within the United States and across the world.[4,5] Its incidence is especially high in South America, affecting 27 per 100,000 people.[6,7] Survival is highly dependent on the stage and depth of tumor invasion. Of all GBC cases, 47% to 70% are discovered incidentally during laparoscopic cholecystectomy or postoperatively on pathologic assessment. Unfortunately, only 40% of incidentally discovered tumors undergo a curative resection.[8]

Surgery alone is the most common treatment modality for GBC (55%) in the United States.[9] Current expert consensus and National Comprehensive Cancer Network guidelines recommend oncologic extended resection (OER) in patients with stage T1b, T2, and T3 GBC with no evidence of disseminated disease. OER includes resection of the gallbladder fossa, dissection of regional lymph nodes, and resection of the common bile duct in selected patients.[10,11] The goals of OER are to allow for accurate staging and, in the case of incidental GBC (IGBC), to remove any residual cancer. Previous studies have shown that residual cancer is found in 38.7% to 61% of patients undergoing OER, and we have reported that the presence of residual cancer is strongly correlated with poor survival, akin to stage IV disease.[3,7,12–15] In contrast, patients with no residual cancer at OER have a 5-year survival rate of up to 85%.[3,13–15]

OER can be performed using the classic open approach or, more recently, minimally invasively. This latter procedure is challenging but can be completed safely and efficiently in expert hands.[16,17] Although laparoscopic liver resection is associated with less bleeding, fewer complications, and a better quality of life than is open resection,[18,19] in cases of GBC, laparoscopic OER is not performed frequently.[20,21] A reason for this is the lack of prospective randomized data, demonstrating the perioperative benefits and oncologic adequacy of laparoscopic OER. We believe that another important factor affecting the adoption of this approach is also the lack of a standardized technique.

In this article, we described a stepwise approach of our experience in laparoscopic OER for GBC.

SURGICAL TECHNIQUE
Preoperative Planning

A preoperative diagnosis of GBC should still be considered a relative contraindication for minimally invasive resection. Patients with large bulky tumors, invasion of the duodenum or colon, and jaundice or hilar involvement are not good candidates for this approach. Ideally, the tumor should be limited to the gallbladder or require less than a major liver resection. In our experience, patients who require a major liver resection for GBC usually have invasion of other organs or proximal bile duct involvement.

Although some patients with IGBC may be good candidates for minimally invasive resection, these cases can be technically challenging. The difficulty of the operation can be estimated using (1) the operative notes from the primary cholecystectomy (a difficult index cholecystectomy will be probably associated with a difficult oncologic resection) and (2) the presence of residual cancer on preoperative imaging, because some of these patients may have invasion of the hepatic pedicle, the duodenum, or the mesocolon. In the preoperative workup, it is crucial that the index cholecystectomy specimen is reviewed again whenever possible by a specialized pathologist assessing the specimen for a positive cystic duct margin, location of the tumor (hepatic vs peritoneal side),[22] perineural and lymphovascular invasion, T status,[3,13–15,23,24] metastasis to cystic duct lymph nodes,[25] and the presence of Rokitansky-Aschoff sinuses,[26] all of which are correlated with the presence of residual cancer. These cases suggest a greater degree of complexity and have a higher chance of needing conversion to open surgery. Therefore, the team performing the OER has to be prepared for conversion.

Preparation and Patient Positioning

The laparoscopic OER can be performed with the patient in a supine position, with the surgeon standing on the right side, or in the French position, with the surgeon standing between the patient's legs. The latter is preferable because the surgeon faces the gallbladder fossa, which allows for a more ergonometric position and optimization of the eye–hand–target–monitor axis. The patient should be securely strapped to the table, because a steep reverse Trendelenburg position and left tilt are usually used. The patient's left arm could be tucked to allow for more space for the surgical assistant(s).

Surgical Approach

The position of the laparoscopic ports is shown in **Fig. 1**. It is our technique to place the optic port in the right upper quadrant, at the mid-clavicle line, which gives an optimal view of the operative field. A 30° optic can be very helpful, especially for the lymph node dissection. For the Pringle maneuver, we prefer a dedicated 5-mm port in the left upper quadrant to not obstruct the field. Other techniques that allow for direct encircling of the hepatic pedicle without using an additional port are available as well. A good way of exposing the gallbladder fossa is by retraction of the round ligament; therefore, we usually mobilize it at the beginning of the operation.

First, it is critical to thoroughly explore the entire abdominal cavity to identify carcinomatosis. Intraoperative ultrasound examination aids in identifying intrahepatic metastases. When operating on a patient with a preoperatively suspected GBC who has not undergone tissue confirmation, this should be done at this step. If there is no visible mass (ie, gallbladder wall thickening or loss of the gallbladder/liver interface), we recommend performing a cholecystectomy and send the specimen for immediate frozen section analysis. This maneuver should be only performed when bile spillage can be avoided. The gallbladder should be removed in a retrieval bag.

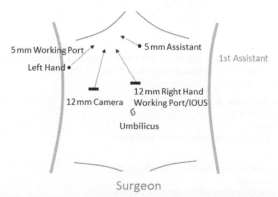

Fig. 1. Port positioning for laparoscopic oncologic extended resection.

SURGICAL PROCEDURE
Step 1: Intercaval–Aortic Node Sampling

Early sampling of the intercaval–aortic nodes (station 16) can allow for a good estimate of the extent of metastatic disease (**Box 1** and Video 1). Very few patients with metastases at this station will derive a benefit from OER and we proceed with OER only in very select patients. The hepatic flexure of the colon in mobilized caudally to fully expose the duodenum. Any omentum that is adherent to the gallbladder fossa should be left in place to be resected en block with the specimen. The peritoneum is incised… over the lateral border of the duodenum and perform a complete Kocher maneuver until the vena cava and aorta are completely exposed. We prefer to not grasp the duodenal wall to avoid injury, but rather gently retract the duodenum anteriorly with a grasper or the aspirator placed behind the head of the pancreas. We recommend starting the lymph node resection caudally on the vena cava side and work your way up to the left renal vein and follow the renal vein to the left until the aorta is exposed. At this point, we can safely complete the dissection on the right border of the aorta. It is important to place clips on any suspected lymph vessel to avoid a postoperative chylous leak. The nodes are then sent for frozen section analysis.

Step 2: Lymph Node Dissection

After the Kocher maneuver, the retropancreatic lymph nodes are exposed. We remove them carefully, taking care not to damage the pancreas, and continue the dissection cranially until we reach lymph node station 12, which is visible on the right side of the junction of the bile duct and the duodenum. At this point, it is easy to identify the portal vein posteriorly. Blunt dissection is used to remove the retroportal lymphatic tissue up to the hepatic hilum.

From the right side of the bile duct, we incise the peritoneum over the superior border of the duodenum to the left and identify the proper hepatic artery. We resect the lymphatic tissue that surrounds the artery from the left border of the bile duct to the left border of the hepatic pedicle. This allows for the retroportal lymph node dissection (station 12p and 12b) to meet with the stations at the left side of the portal vein (station 12a and 5). From here, we extend the dissection up to the hepatic hilum.

Box 1
Gallbladder cancer: laparoscopic oncologic resection

Step 1: Intercaval–aortic node sampling
- Expose duodenum and perform the Kocher maneuver
- Lymphadenectomy from caudal to cranial and from right to left
- Prevent chyle leaks

Step 2: Lymph node dissection
- Be systematic: retropancreatic > retroportal > hepatic pedicle > common hepatic artery
- Limited dissection around the common bile duct to avoid injury
- Optimal hemostasis is critical

Step 3: Resection of the cystic duct
- Identification: look for clips
- Avoid energy devices
- Dissect the duct up to the insertion in the bile duct

Step 4: Liver resection
- For most cases, a 2-cm wedge resection is adequate
- Use the Pringle maneuver
- Anticipate the distal branches of the middle hepatic vein

You should be able to identify the left and right hepatic arteries. Extended dissection over the bile duct should be avoided, otherwise, its blood supply could be seriously compromised leading to strictures.

From the proper hepatic artery, we identify the common hepatic artery and incise the peritoneum over the superior border of the body of the pancreas. Then we resect the anterosuperior lymphatic tissue surrounding the common hepatic artery (stations 5 and 8). We take time to control the small arterial branches near the pancreas as well as the left gastric vein. The portal vein here is superficial, just under the peritoneum of the left border of the hepatic pedicle, hidden behind the common hepatic artery. Care must be taken not to damage it. Blunt dissection is useful.

Step 3: Resection of the Cystic Duct in Patients with incidental gallbladder cancer

Resection of the cystic duct is a commonly overlooked step, but it is very important because it may change the planned operation (ie, resection of the bile duct) and affect prognosis (Video 2). The most difficult aspect of this procedure is the accurate identification of the cystic duct. The operative notes from the index cholecystectomy and the results of the pathologic assessment of the cholecystectomy specimen can be very helpful. Metallic clips on the right side of the bile duct or at the base of the gallbladder fossa can be a telltale sign for locating the cystic duct. We recommend carefully dissecting the tissue around the clips with scissors rather than an energy device to avoid a heat injury to the bile duct. To determine the precise status of the cystic duct, it should be dissected up to the insertion on the bile duct and sent for frozen section analysis. Nevertheless, in a substantial number of cases a cystic duct cannot be easily identified and overly aggressive dissection at this step to identify a stump should be avoided to prevent a common bile duct injury.

Step 4: Liver Resection

It is rare that a major hepatectomy for GBC becomes necessary (Video 3). Resection of the gallbladder fossa is the objective in this case, and the extent of hepatectomy varies between excision of the gallbladder fossa to anatomic segment 4b/5 resection; however, there are no clear data to support one method over the other. In patients with IGBC, we believe that at least a 2-cm resection of the gallbladder fossa is required.

We always use the Pringle maneuver to minimize bleeding and keep the field clean, which allows for a quicker and safer resection. A simple method of performing this maneuver is to pass a small feeding tube around the hepatic pedicle and attach it snugly with a piece of tubular drain using a grasper and a dedicated 5-mm port. Another way is to use a laparoscopic vascular clamp. The occlusion can be kept safely on for 15 to 20 minutes and can be repeated several times throughout the procedure, with 5- to 10-minute recovery times in between.

After marking the liver capsule for the parenchymal transection line around the gallbladder fossa, we place stay sutures at the borders of the specimen; these sutures are very useful for traction and mobilization of the often fragile liver specimen. We perform the liver resection in a crush/clamp technique using the energy device (bipolar forceps and harmonic scalpel). It is important to identify the distal middle hepatic vein branches (V5 and V4b) at the level of the gallbladder fossa, which can be a major source of bleeding during the transection.

Step 5: Extraction and Final Revision

We extract the specimen in a retrieval bag through a slightly enlarged port site or a small transverse suprapubic incision. In our practice, we always leave a drain.

At the end of the operation, we systemically inspect to operative field for potential areas of complications.

1. Bleeding
    • Intercaval–aortic dissection
    • Retropancreatic dissection
    • Common hepatic artery dissection
    • Liver transection
2. Leaks
    • Liver transection for bile
    • Intercaval–aortic area for chyle (Video 4)

SHORT- AND LONG-TERM OUTCOMES

The published series of laparoscopic OER are relatively recent (**Table 1**) and show similar perioperative outcomes between them. Operative times and blood loss reflect the usual learning curve issues observed for other new laparoscopic procedures. Perioperative outcomes for complex laparoscopic procedures have been addressed in high-quality prospective studies for liver resections, colon and gastric cancer,[19,27,28] and recent reports of laparoscopic OER (see **Table 1**) show promising early outcomes. In contrast, because there are only a few nonrandomized comparative reports of laparoscopic versus open surgery available,[29,30] oncologic long-term adequacy of laparoscopic surgery for GBC remains to be further investigated and should, therefore, be performed only in selected centers with experience in GBC and laparoscopic surgery.

When we compared our experience of 35 patients who underwent laparoscopic approach with a matched historical cohort of open cases,[31] we found that a positive liver margin at time of the index cholecystectomy and an interval between surgeries of more than 60 days were predictive for conversion to open surgery. Blood loss, operative time, number and positive lymph nodes, R1 disease, residual cancer, overall morbidity, Clavien grade III, 90-day mortality, and recurrence patterns were comparable. Similar to previous reports,[30] the median hospital stay for laparoscopic OER was significant shorter compared with an open approach (4 days vs 6 days; $P = .032$).

Accurate prognosis for GBC is related to optimal lymph node staging. This staging can be achieved with a systematic and complete dissection, as we have described. In our experience, the median number of lymph nodes retrieved is the same as in open OER (6 lymph nodes). This is crucial because, in the 8th edition of the American Joint Committee on Cancer, the number of lymph nodes analyzed dictates the nodal category.[32] It is recommended that at least 6 lymph nodes be harvested and evaluated[33,34] during the OER.

Although there are few data on long-term survival, most reports in the literature show comparable survival rates between laparoscopic OER and open OER.[29–31,34,35] Yoon and colleagues[35] showed that the 5-year disease specific survival rate was 94.2% in a group of 45 selected stage T1 to T2 patients. Other study[30] compared 16 stage T2 patients that had a laparoscopic OER with 14 patients (T stage not specified) open and showed no statistically significant difference in either the disease-free survival or overall survival rate between the groups, although there was a tendency toward less recurrence and better survival in the laparoscopic group, which may have to do with selection bias. Interestingly, there was no recurrence in the laparoscopic group after a mean follow-up of 37 months.

When attempting to manage the challenging disease of GBC minimally invasively, great care must be taken to meet the standard of care. First, the current experience in laparoscopic OER apply mainly to patients requiring gallbladder bed resection

Table 1
Laparoscopic radical cholecystectomy series to date

Factors	Cho et al,[37] 2010	de Aretxabala et al,[40] 2010	Shen et al,[38] 2012	Gumbs et al,[39] 2013	Itano et al,[35] 2015	Yoon et al,[30] 2015	Agarwal et al,[29] 2015	Shirobe and Maruyama,[41] 2015	Palanisamy et al,[42] 2016
Study period	2004–2007	2005–2009	2010–2011	2005–2011	2007–2013	2004–2014	2011–2013	2001–2013	2008–2013
Control group, open surgery	No	No	No	No	Yes	No	Yes	No	No
Number of patients	18	7	5	15	16	32	24	11, only 6 cases liver bed resection	12
Inclusion of non-IGBC	Yes	Yes	Yes	Yes	Yes	Yes	Yes	Yes	Yes
Inclusion of T3 stage	No	Yes	Yes	Yes	No	No	Yes	No	Yes
Intraoperative ultrasound examination	Yes	Yes		Yes	Yes	Yes	NR	No	NR
Conversion to open procedure	4 (22)	10	0	1	0	1	NR	0	0
Intraoperative bleeding accident	1	NR				1	0	0	0
Intraoperative bile duct injury	1	NR		NR	NR	1	NR	0	0
Lymph node yield	8 (4–21)	6 (3–12)	9 (3–11)	4 (1–11)	12.6 SD-3.1	7 (1–15)	10 (4–31)	13 (9–18)	8 (4–14)
Aortocaval sampling	No	Yes	No	Yes	No	No	Yes	No	No
Operative time, min	190 (90-277)	NR	200 (120–300)	220 (120–480)	368 SD 73	205 (90–360)	270 (180–340)	196 (149–490)	213 SD 27
Operative blood loss, mL	50 (10-400)	NR	210 (50–400)	160 (0–400)	152 SD-90	100 (10–1500)	200 (100–850)	92 (10–643)	196 SD 63

(continued on next page)

Table 1
(continued)

Factors	Cho et al,[37] 2010	de Aretxabala et al,[40] 2010	Shen et al,[38] 2012	Gumbs et al,[39] 2013	Itano et al,[30] 2015	Yoon et al,[35] 2015	Agarwal et al,[29] 2015	Shirobe and Maruyama,[41] 2015	Palanisamy et al,[42] 2016
Common bile duct resection	No	0	0	2	0	0	0	1	0
R1 patients	NR	0	NR	0	NR	0	0	2	0
Morbidity	3	0	0	0	1	6	3	1	3
Clavien ≥3	1	0	0	0	0	2	NR	0	1
Bile leak	1	0	0	0	0	0	2	0	2
Postoperative bleeding, collection	0	0	0	0	0	0	1	0	0
Length of stay, days	4 (3–11)	3	7 (7–8)	4 (2–8)	9.1 SD-1.6	4 (2–13)	5 (3–16)	6 (4–19)	5 SD 1
30-Day mortality	NR	0	0	0	0	0	0	0	0
Follow-up, months	27 (15–57)	22	11 (1–17)	23 (9–38)	37	60 (3.5–118.9)[a]	18 (6–34)	93 (13–152)	51 (14–70)
Recurrence	0	1	1 (20)	2 (13)	0	4 (8.9)[a]	1 (4)	2	3 (25)

Abbreviations: IGBC, incidental gallbladder cancer; NR, not reported; R1, microscopic positive margin; SD, standard deviation.
[a] Including 13 open surgery patients.

and lymphadenectomy, excluding patients with extensive bile duct and adjacent organs involvement. Second, although patients should have general access to the reduced morbidity of minimally invasive management of GBC, we believed that the learning curve for minimally invasive surgery for GBC should be undertaken in specialized hepatobiliary units with appropriate case volume, experience in open and minimally invasive hepatobiliary surgery, and infrastructural commitment to developing this approach. Third, it is important to understand that this minimally invasive technique is an option for select surgeons with special expertise in managing GBC and performing advanced laparoscopic surgery. A wise selection should be based on a thoughtful review of the operative notes and pathologic specimen of the index cholecystectomy, whenever available, looking for technical difficulties or high risk prognostic factors,[3,12–15,22–25] serologic makers as CA19-9,[36] and abdominal imaging as ultrasound and computed tomography scans. All of these considerations should guide the need for additional workup to optimize patient selection for minimally invasive management of GBC.

CLINICAL RESULTS IN THE LITERATURE

Table 1 presents clinical results found in the literature.

SUMMARY

Minimally invasive OER for selected patients with GBC should be performed in a systematic and stepwise approach in centers with experience in open OER. In experienced hands, laparoscopic resection can be performed safely with excellent perioperative outcomes and decreased morbidity compared with an open approach. Minimally invasive management of GBC mainly applies to patients with early GBC or IGBC. Long-term survival seems to be similar to open surgery, although more data are needed to confirm these results. Dissemination of advanced laparoscopic skills and a timely referral of GBC patients to specialized centers may allow more patients to benefit from this less invasive operation.

ACKNOWLEDGEMENTS

The authors thank Ann M. Sutton, Department of Scientific Publications at MD Anderson Cancer Center, for copyediting the manuscript.

SUPPLEMENTARY DATA

Supplementary data related to this article can be found online at https://doi.org/10.1016/j.soc.2018.11.001.

REFERENCES

1. Henley SJ, Weir HK, Jim MA, et al. Gallbladder cancer incidence and mortality, United States 1999-2011. Cancer Epidemiol Biomarkers Prev 2015;24(9): 1319–26.
2. Hundal R, Shaffer EA. Gallbladder cancer: epidemiology and outcome. Clin Epidemiol 2014;6:99–109.
3. Vinuela E, Vega EA, Yamashita S, et al. Incidental gallbladder cancer: residual cancer discovered at oncologic extended resection determines outcome: a report from high- and low-incidence countries. Ann Surg Oncol 2017;24(8):2334–43.

4. Butte JM, Torres J, Veras EF, et al. Regional differences in gallbladder cancer pathogenesis: insights from a comparison of cell cycle-regulatory, PI3K, and pro-angiogenic protein expression. Ann Surg Oncol 2013;20(5):1470–81.
5. Butte JM, Matsuo K, Gonen M, et al. Gallbladder cancer: differences in presentation, surgical treatment, and survival in patients treated at centers in three countries. J Am Coll Surg 2011;212(1):50–61.
6. Lazcano-Ponce EC, Miquel JF, Munoz N, et al. Epidemiology and molecular pathology of gallbladder cancer. CA Cancer J Clin 2001;51(6):349–64.
7. Butte JM, Waugh E, Meneses M, et al. Incidental gallbladder cancer: analysis of surgical findings and survival. J Surg Oncol 2010;102(6):620–5.
8. Duffy A, Capanu M, Abou-Alfa GK, et al. Gallbladder cancer (GBC): 10-year experience at Memorial Sloan-Kettering Cancer Centre (MSKCC). J Surg Oncol 2008;98(7):485–9.
9. Lau CSM, Zywot A, Mahendraraj K, et al. Gallbladder Carcinoma in the United States: a population based clinical outcomes study involving 22,343 patients from the surveillance, epidemiology, and end result database (1973-2013). HPB Surg 2017;2017:1532835.
10. Benson AB 3rd, Abrams TA, Ben-Josef E, et al. NCCN clinical practice guidelines in oncology: hepatobiliary cancers. J Natl Compr Canc Netw 2009;7(4):350–91.
11. Aloia TA, Jarufe N, Javle M, et al. Gallbladder cancer: expert consensus statement. HPB (Oxford) 2015;17(8):681–90.
12. Choi KS, Choi SB, Park P, et al. Clinical characteristics of incidental or unsuspected gallbladder cancers diagnosed during or after cholecystectomy: a systematic review and meta-analysis. World J Gastroenterol 2015;21(4):1315–23.
13. Butte JM, Kingham TP, Gonen M, et al. Residual disease predicts outcomes after definitive resection for incidental gallbladder cancer. J Am Coll Surg 2014;219(3):416–29.
14. Lendoire JC, Gil L, Duek F, et al. Relevance of residual disease after liver resection for incidental gallbladder cancer. HPB (Oxford) 2012;14(8):548–53.
15. Pawlik TM, Gleisner AL, Vigano L, et al. Incidence of finding residual disease for incidental gallbladder carcinoma: implications for re-resection. J Gastrointest Surg 2007;11(11):1478–86 [discussion: 1486–7].
16. Vega EA, Yamashita S, Chun YS, et al. Effective laparoscopic management lymph node dissection for gallbladder cancer. Ann Surg Oncol 2017;24(7):1852.
17. Yamashita S, Loyer E, Chun YS, et al. Laparoscopic management of gallbladder cancer: a stepwise approach. Ann Surg Oncol 2016;23(Suppl 5):892–3.
18. Nguyen KT, Gamblin TC, Geller DA. World review of laparoscopic liver resection-2,804 patients. Ann Surg 2009;250(5):831–41.
19. Fretland AA, Dagenborg VJ, Bjornelv GMW, et al. Laparoscopic versus open resection for colorectal liver metastases: the OSLO-COMET randomized controlled trial. Ann Surg 2018;267(2):199–207.
20. Machado MA, Makdissi FF, Surjan RC. Totally laparoscopic hepatic bisegmentectomy (s4b+s5) and hilar lymphadenectomy for incidental gallbladder cancer. Ann Surg Oncol 2015;22(Suppl 3):S336–9.
21. Gumbs AA, Hoffman JP. Laparoscopic completion radical cholecystectomy for T2 gallbladder cancer. Surg Endosc 2010;24(12):3221–3.
22. Shindoh J, de Aretxabala X, Aloia TA, et al. Tumor location is a strong predictor of tumor progression and survival in T2 gallbladder cancer: an international multicenter study. Ann Surg 2015;261(4):733–9.
23. Ethun CG, Postlewait LM, Le N, et al. A novel pathology-based preoperative risk score to predict locoregional residual and distant disease and survival for

incidental gallbladder cancer: a 10-institution study from the U.S. extrahepatic biliary malignancy consortium. Ann Surg Oncol 2017;24(5):1343–50.

24. Creasy JM, Goldman DA, Gonen M, et al. Predicting residual disease in incidental gallbladder cancer: risk stratification for modified treatment strategies. J Gastrointest Surg 2017;21(8):1254–61.

25. Vega EA, Vinuela E, Yamashita S, et al. Extended lymphadenectomy is required for incidental gallbladder cancer independent of cystic duct lymph node status. J Gastrointest Surg 2018;22(1):43–51.

26. Roa JC, Tapia O, Manterola C, et al. Early gallbladder carcinoma has a favorable outcome but Rokitansky-Aschoff sinus involvement is an adverse prognostic factor. Virchows Arch 2013;463(5):651–61.

27. Kim YW, Yoon HM, Yun YH, et al. Long-term outcomes of laparoscopy-assisted distal gastrectomy for early gastric cancer: result of a randomized controlled trial (COACT 0301). Surg Endosc 2013;27(11):4267–76.

28. Lacy AM, Garcia-Valdecasas JC, Delgado S, et al. Laparoscopy-assisted colectomy versus open colectomy for treatment of non-metastatic colon cancer: a randomised trial. Lancet 2002;359(9325):2224–9.

29. Agarwal AK, Javed A, Kalayarasan R, et al. Minimally invasive versus the conventional open surgical approach of a radical cholecystectomy for gallbladder cancer: a retrospective comparative study. HPB (Oxford) 2015;17(6):536–41.

30. Itano O, Oshima G, Minagawa T, et al. Novel strategy for laparoscopic treatment of pT2 gallbladder carcinoma. Surg Endosc 2015;29(12):3600–7.

31. Vega EA, De Arextabala X, Okuno M, et al. Safe laparoscopic oncologic resection of incidentally discovered gallbladder cancer: a propensity score matching analysis. In. Abstract. 13th IHPBA. Geneva, Switzerland, September 4-7, 2018.

32. Sakata J, Shirai Y, Wakai T, et al. Number of positive lymph nodes independently determines the prognosis after resection in patients with gallbladder carcinoma. Ann Surg Oncol 2010;17(7):1831–40.

33. Liu GJ, Li XH, Chen YX, et al. Radical lymph node dissection and assessment: impact on gallbladder cancer prognosis. World J Gastroenterol 2013;19(31):5150–8.

34. Ito H, Ito K, D'Angelica M, et al. Accurate staging for gallbladder cancer: implications for surgical therapy and pathological assessment. Ann Surg 2011; 254(2):320–5.

35. Yoon YS, Han HS, Cho JY, et al. Is laparoscopy contraindicated for gallbladder cancer? a 10-year prospective Cohort Study. J Am Coll Surg 2015;221(4):847–53.

36. Yamashita S, Passot G, Aloia TA, et al. Prognostic value of carbohydrate antigen 19-9 in patients undergoing resection of biliary tract cancer. Br J Surg 2017; 104(3):267–77.

37. Cho JY, Han HS, Yoon YS, et al. Laparoscopic approach for suspected early-stage gallbladder carcinoma. Arch Surg 2010;145(2):128–33.

38. Shen BY, Zhan Q, Deng XX, et al. Radical resection of gallbladder cancer: could it be robotic? Surg Endosc 2012;26(11):3245–50.

39. Gumbs AA, Jarufe N, Gayet B. Minimally invasive approaches to extrapancreatic cholangiocarcinoma. Surg Endosc 2013;27(2):406–14.

40. de Aretxabala X, Leon J, Hepp J, et al. Gallbladder cancer: role of laparoscopy in the management of potentially resectable tumors. Surg Endosc 2010;24(9):2192–6.

41. Shirobe T, Maruyama S. Laparoscopic radical cholecystectomy with lymph node dissection for gallbladder carcinoma. Surg Endosc 2015;29(8):2244–50.

42. Palanisamy S, Patel N, Sabnis S, et al. Laparoscopic radical cholecystectomy for suspected early gall bladder carcinoma: thinking beyond convention. Surg Endosc 2016;30(6):2442–8.

Minimally Invasive Approaches to Pancreatic Cancer

Joseph R. Broucek, MD[a,b,*], Dominic Sanford, MD[b,c],
John A. Stauffer, MD[b], Horacio J. Asbun, MD[b,d,e]

KEYWORDS

- Laparoscopic whipple • Minimally invasive whipple
- Minimally invasive pancreaticoduodenectomy • Pancreas
- Minimally invasive surgery

KEY POINTS

- Minimally invasive approaches to pancreatic cancer are technically feasible with appropriate training after a learning curve.
- Review of the steps of the most common minimally invasive operations is summarized in this article.
- Minimally invasive surgery in treating pancreatic cancer has comparable oncologic outcomes for the patient.
- The cost of implementing these techniques in treating pancreatic cancer is comparable to traditional approaches when factoring in morbidity and length of stay for high-volume institutions.
- A review of the literature demonstrates comparable outcomes of morbidity and mortality as well as long-term survival for pancreatic cancer.

Pancreatic cancer has been at the center of an ongoing crusade to discovery of improved means of care. Pancreatic adenocarcinoma maintains an increasing incidence since the 1990s for many known and unknown reasons. Despite improvement in neoadjuvant therapy, adjuvant therapy, and diagnostics, the mortality remains unchanged as the fourth leading cause of cancer death in the United States with more

Disclosure Statement: No disclosures.
[a] Department of Surgery, Vanderbilt University Medical Center, 1161 21st Avenue South, D5203 MCN, Nashville, TN 37232, USA; [b] Department of General Surgery, Mayo Clinic, Davis 3N, 4500 San Pablo Road, Jacksonville, FL 32224, USA; [c] Department of Surgery, Washington University School of Medicine, Barnes-Jewish Hospital, 1 Barnes Jewish Hospital Plaza, St. Louis, MO 63110, USA; [d] Miami Cancer Institute, 8900 North Kendall Drive, Miami, FL 33176, USA; [e] Mayo Clinic College of Medicine and Sciences, 200 First Street South West, Rochester, MN 55905, USA
* Corresponding author. 1161 21st Avenue South, Room D5203 MCN, Nashville, TN 37232.
E-mail address: joebroucek@gmail.com

than 30,000 deaths per year.[1–3] Pancreatic resection combined with neoadjuvant and/ or adjuvant therapy remains the only chance for cure and/or prolonged survival. Surgical resection is associated with a significant morbidity ranging from 30% to 60%, and with mortality in the range of 1% to 17%.[4–6]

In recent years, a minimally invasive approach to pancreatic cancer has gained increased acceptance and popularity. The role of minimally invasive surgery in pancreatic cancer has been previously limited to diagnostic laparoscopy to rule out occult lesions in the liver and peritoneum in order to avoid unnecessary laparotomy and resection. The advent of laparoscopy and distal pancreatectomy began with Soper and colleagues[7] in 1994, and, currently, has shown improved results when compared with an open approach.[8,9] Expansion to right-sided pancreatic resection has gained acceptance only as of recent despite its first human description being in the mid 1990s.[6,10] The aim of minimally invasive surgery of the pancreas is similar to all other approaches to minimally invasive oncologic surgery, including limiting abdominal trauma, decreasing length of hospitalization, decreasing overall cost, decreasing blood loss, allowing for a more meticulous oncologic dissection, and overall aiming for a better operation.

As recommended in open pancreatic surgery, the surgeon's focused training and experience in pancreas surgery are of utmost importance to transition to a minimally invasive approach.[5,6,11,12] New advances in technology, including advanced endoscopic skills and routine use in practice, have helped progress in this field. Furthermore, 3-dimensional endoscopic tools and the introduction of robotics have made the minimally invasive approach more feasible among surgeons at various levels in the learning curve. In this article, the minimally invasive surgical approaches to proximal, central, and distal pancreatic cancer are described.

RIGHT-SIDED PANCREATIC RESECTION

As with most carcinomas, right-sided pancreatic cancer resections are taken on with an R0 intent, requiring intense focus on complete and clear dissection from vascular structures and surrounding local tissue. Total mobilization and clearance of tissue from around the superior mesenteric vein (SMV), portal vein (PV), superior mesenteric artery, and other local vascular structures are critical. Furthermore, partial or complete resection and reconstruction of the SMV and/or PV may be needed to achieve R0 resection.[1] In order to take on the challenges of laparoscopic pancreaticoduodenectomy (LPD), the surgeon(s) must preferably have extensive experience with an open approach or specific training, have a focus in MIS pancreas surgery, have a willingness to withstand a major time commitment during the learning curve, and have access to the necessary equipment to make such an undertaking feasible.[12]

Technique

The patient is placed in a supine split-leg position allowing the operating surgeon and assistants to switch positions based on the portion of the procedure that is being performed. In this technique, anywhere from 4 to 7 trocars are used. In the authors' practice, they use a 6-trocar approach that is positioned in a semicircle fashion around the head of the pancreas (**Fig. 1**). Four of the trocars are 10 to 12 mm in order to allow for frequent repositioning of the camera, linear stapler, and other larger instruments throughout the case based on the stage of the operation and position of the operating surgeon.

The camera is inserted, and metastatic or obvious unresectable disease is ruled out. Attention is first paid to entering the lesser sac and mobilizing the greater curvature of the stomach toward the duodenum. A pyloric-preserving procedure is performed and,

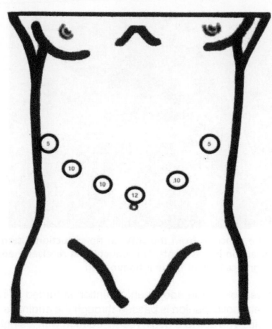

Fig. 1. Trocar placement for an LPD. (*Courtesy of* the Mayo Foundation for Medical Education and Research. All rights reserved; with permission.)

as such, careful attention is paid to preserve the gastroepiploic artery. The hepatic flexure and transverse colon are mobilized, including part of the ascending colon. The patient is positioned in the reverse Trendelenburg to allow for gravity retraction of the colon. The first portion of the duodenum is surrounded in 360° at approximately 3 cm distal to the pylorus, stapled, and divided. Next, the hepatic artery is exposed. The station 8A lymph node is excised, and the hepatic artery is traced to the gastro-duodenal artery, which is then also dissected and ligated. The common bile duct is dissected circumferentially and sharply divided leaving the posterior wall longer than the anterior, which facilitates reconstruction. A bulldog clamp is placed on the common bile duct to prevent any further spillage. Vascular control of the PV with placement of a vessel loop may be performed at this time as well if needed. Attention is focused at the inferior aspect of the neck of the pancreas, where the SMV is identified, and again vascular control may be achieved with a vessel loop if vascular resection is a possibility. The pancreas is then separated from the superior mesenteric-PV trunk, and a band-passer is used to place a Penrose drain around the pancreas to aid in retraction. The pancreatic parenchyma is divided with ultrasonic shears until the main pancreatic duct is identified, which is cut with cold scissors approximately 2 to 3 mm to the patient's right of the pancreas allowing for a small protruding stump for reconstruction (**Fig. 2**). The camera is moved one trocar to the right, when previously it was in the center. Focus is now on performing a wide Kocherization of the duodenum, which is further facilitated by using the assistant to the patient's left to caudally retract the mobilized right and transverse colon inferiorly and the duodenal stump cranially. A wide Kocher maneuver allows for harvesting of the retroperitoneal/retropancreatic and retrocholedochal lymph nodes. The uncinated process is then meticulously separated from the SMV and artery, allowing for a complete neuro-lymphatic clearance. If necessary, partial or resection of the superior mesenteric/PV can be performed depending on surgeon experience.

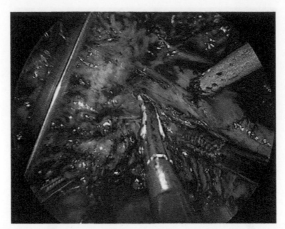

Fig. 2. Dissection of the pancreas from the SMV (at tip of suction) using a bipolar energy device and critical retraction by assistants. This patient had received neoadjuvant therapy, which often creates significant local tissue inflammation.

After complete resection of the specimen, attention is turned to reconstruction. A limb of jejunum in a retrocolic fashion is passed through the original extended opening of the ligament of Treitz. The authors begin reconstruction with a single-layer choledo-chojejunostomy using a running absorbable braided suture (**Figs. 3** and **4**). They then perform a 2-layer pancreaticojejunostomy (**Figs. 5** and **6**). A nonabsorbable monofilament suture is used for the outer layers. A 5-0 braided absorbable suture on an ophthalmologic needle is used for the inner duct-to-mucosal layer in an interrupted fashion. The gastrointestinal reconstruction is done by creating a duodenojejunostomy in a 2-layer end-to-side fashion with an antecolic loop of small bowel (**Figs. 7** and **8**). The pylorus is dilated before completing the inner layer with a laparoscopic debakey. The specimen is oriented for extraction and extracted via the periumbilical port site, which is extended to the smallest size that would allow extraction.

Outcomes of Right-Sided Pancreatectomy

There are numerous published outcomes regarding the safety and feasibility of mini-mally invasive pancreaticoduodenectomy in the hands of technically experienced

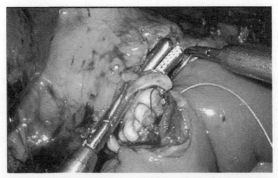

Fig. 3. Creation of the choledochojejunostomy. The posterior wall anastomosis is shown. Leaving the posterior common bile duct wall longer than the anterior wall during division allows for more ease during the choledochojejunostomy.

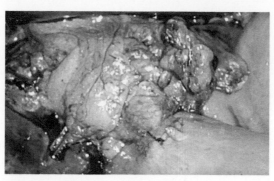

Fig. 4. The completed choledochojejunostomy.

surgeons.[13] The National Cancer Database was reviewed by Adam and colleagues[6] and identified 7061 pancreaticoduodenectomy cases from 2010 to 2011 with 14% (983) performed via a minimally invasive approach and the remaining 86% performed open pancreaticoduodenectomy (OPD) (conversion rate of 30%). Interestingly, 92% of the 144 hospitals performing LPD did 10 or less cases a year with only half performing only 1 LPD. Based on this review, the unadjusted 30-day mortality after a minimally invasive approach was 4.8% versus 3.7% in the open group ($P = .10$). There was no difference in lymph node retrieval number, positive margin rate, length of stay, or 30-day unplanned readmission rates. This review is limited because most of these cases were performed at low-volume centers. The aforementioned data is supported by Doula and colleagues,[14] who reviewed 14 other high-yield single-institution series that showed no differences in resection margins, fistula formation, bile leak, delayed gastric emptying, reoperation rates, or mortality. Again, blood loss was less with the minimally invasive approach.

A large series of LPD published at a single high-volume institution was performed by Croome and colleagues[15] at the Mayo Clinic–Rochester. They compared 108 LPDs with 214 OPDs. The laparoscopic group was associated with a 3-day shorter hospitalization and a quicker return to chemotherapy than the open group. Furthermore, they showed that a laparoscopic approach had a lower rate of delayed gastric emptying compared with in the open group. All cases were pyloric preserving in technique. The authors' group at the Mayo Clinic–Florida published their series of 58 LPD versus

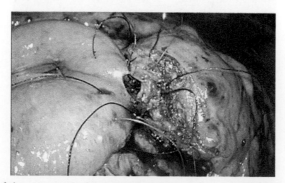

Fig. 5. Creation of the pancreaticojejunostomy using a 5-0 nonabsorbable monofilament suture for the outer layers. A 5-0 braided absorbable suture on an ophthalmologic needle is used for the inner duct-to-mucosal layer in an interrupted fashion.

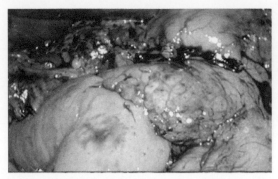

Fig. 6. The completed pancreaticojejunostomy.

193 open procedures. They again showed a hospital length of stay of 3 days less in the laparoscopic group (6 vs 9 days) and a shorter duration to chemotherapy. Blood loss was less in LPD at 250 mL versus 600 mL in the open group, resulting in fewer transfusions. In addition, LPD was associated with greater lymph node harvest (27 vs 17 nodes). There was no difference in morbidity or mortality emphasizing the safety of this technique.[16] Although the National Cancer Database did not show any improvement in morbidity or mortality in the laparoscopic approach, Hyder and colleagues[5] reported a 10% lower rate of mortality at high-volume centers (more than 25 cases/y) compared with centers that performed less than 4 cases per year.[1] One report on long-term oncologic safety of the LPD was by Conrad and colleagues[17] in 2017. Their article looked at 1-, 3-, and 5-year overall survival and recurrence-free survival (40 LPD and 25 OPD patients). At 5 years, overall survival was 35.5 versus 29.6 months ($P = .25$). Recurrence-free survival was 21.9% versus 25.7% at 5 years ($P = .39$, LPD vs OPD). Complications such as pancreatic fistula rate, delayed gastric emptying, bile leak, hemorrhage, reoperation, and mortality are also comparable in LPD versus OPD.[17] What this shows is that LPD is noninferior to OPD regarding oncologic outcomes and overall morbidity/mortality at 5 years for patients with adenocarcinoma. **Table 1** summarizes the major meta-analyses comparing open and minimally invasive pancreaticoduodenectomy.[18–27]

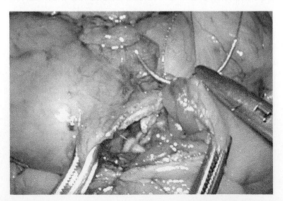

Fig. 7. The gastrointestinal reconstruction is done by creating a duodenojejunostomy in a 2-layer end-to-side fashion with an antecolic loop of small bowel. The back wall and transition to front wall anastomosis is shown.

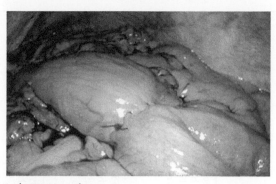

Fig. 8. The completed anastomosis.

When adopting new technologies in a hospital system, cost is of course a concern. Several studies have looked at this; however, it is a challenge as to how to assess overall cost to the hospital system and society. Although it is a bit easier to examine cost at an institutional level, there are other factors, such as quality of life, postoperative events, and ability to return to work, that need further evaluation. At the Mayo Clinic–Florida, a cost analysis of open versus LPD was performed.[28] The authors' cost analysis included the use of the hospital billing database to look at surgical costs, including operating room (OR) time and surgical supplies, admission costs, and overall cost of care during index admission. Forty-eight OPD and 75 LPD patients were compared having equal morbidity, age, gender, American Society of Anesthesiologists airway grade, rates of vein resection, and indication for surgery. The authors' data showed that LPD had higher surgical costs due to increased OR time and surgical supply utility. However, OPD was associated with higher hospital admission costs that then offset overall cost, making both techniques equivalent. Gerber and colleagues[29] further support these data in their study of 52 LPD versus 50 OPD patients. Total OR costs were $12,290 for LPD versus $11,299 dollars for OPD ($P = .05$) attributed to added supply cost in the LPD group. Although length of stay was shorter in the LPD group (both OPD and LPD underwent an Enhanced recovery after surgery [ERAS] protocol), overall index hospitalization cost was $28,496 in the LPD group and $28,623 in the OPD group. Surgically related readmissions and cost did not differ between the 2 groups; however, fewer patients required discharge to a skill facility after index hospitalization (88% in the OPD group vs 72%, $P = .047$), which suggests that overall cost, including postoperative discharge and care, is likely less in the LPD group.

What these data show, most importantly, is that there is proven evidence of lower rates of blood loss and length of hospital stay, return to diet, and quicker return to chemotherapy postoperatively without compromising oncologic outcomes.[6,15,16,30] Furthermore, cost to the institution in experienced hands is, at least, equivalent. It is quite evident that the minimally invasive approach to right-sided pancreatic tumors is gaining interest and popularity among hospitals across the United States and the globe. However, one should emphasize that the studies appear to show lesser quality outcomes in low-volume centers.

DISTAL PANCREATIC RESECTION

Laparoscopic distal pancreatectomy (LDP), as stated earlier, was first discussed by Soper and colleagues[7] in 1994 in the porcine model, and the first reported case performed in a human was by Gagner and Pomp[10] in the mid 1990s. Since then, many

Table 1
Meta-analyses comparing open and minimally invasive pancreaticoduodenectomy

Reference/ No. of Studies	No. of Patients (Open/MIS PD)	EBL	Operative Time	POPF/Overall Complications	LOS	Margins	Nodes	Conclusions
Correa-Gallego et al,[18] 2014	373/169	Less with MIS PD WMD 1460 mL P<.001	Longer with MIS PD WMD 131 min P = .003	No significant difference POPF 21% MIS vs 17% OPD P = .94/.15	Shorter with MIS PD 3.7 d less P = .02	Lower R1 margins for MIS PD P = .007	Increased lymph node harvest for MIS PD 3 nodes more P = .03	MIS PD is feasible, associated with improved outcomes but superiority cannot be confirmed without RCTs
Nigri et al,[19] 2014	419/204	Less with MIS PD P<.0001	Longer with MIS PD P<.0001	No significant difference P = .80/.34	Shorter with MIS PD P = .0497	Lower R1 margins for MIS PD P = .90	Increased lymph node harvest for MIS PD P = .050	MIS PD is safe and feasible in expert hands, may reduce overall complications similar POPF, DGE
Qin et al,[20] 2014	542/327	Less with MIS PD MD −362 mL P<.001	Longer with MIS PD MD 105 min P<.001	No significant difference P = .86/.05	Shorter with MIS PD WMD −2.6 d P = .001	Similar R0 margins P = .07	Similar lymph node harvest P = .48	MIS PD associated with some advantages, should be performed in high-volume institute in patient with minimal pancreatitis and small cancers

Study								
Lei et al,[21] 2014	429/209	Less with MIS PD WMD −406 mL P = .007	Longer with MIS PD WMD 107 min P = .007	No significant difference P = .78/.16	Shorter with MIS PD WMD −4.14 d P = .02	Lower R1 margins for MIS PD P = .03	Similar lymph node harvest P = .11	MIS PD is feasible, likely with improved outcomes. Selection bias had minimal effect on final outcomes
de Rooij et al,[22] 2016	26,131/2759	Less with MIS PD WMD −385 mL P = .001	Longer with MIS PD WMD 73.5 min P = .001	No significant difference P = .0009/NR	Shorter with MIS PD WMD −3.1 d P<.0001	Lower R1 margins for MIS PD P = .04	Similar lymph node harvest P = .76	MIS PD with some advantages, should be practiced in high volume centers with a structured training program
Zhang et al,[23] 2016	5102/1018	Less with MIS PD WMD −312 mL P<.001	Longer with MIS PD WMD 83.9 min P<.001	No significant difference P = .17/.86	Shorter with MIS PD WMD −3.57 P<.001	Lower R1 margins for MIS PD P<.001	Increased lymph node harvest with MIS PD P<.001	MIS PD can be a reasonable alternative to OPD with potential advantages
Wang et al,[24] 2017	1306/1603	Less with MIS PD WMD −300 mL P<.0001	Longer with MIS PD WMD 71 min P = .002	No significant difference P = .30/NR	Shorter with MIS PD WMD −2.95 P<.0001	Lower R1 margins for MIS PD P = .0003	Increased lymph node harvest with MIS PD P = .03	MIS PD is safe, feasible, and worthwhile

(continued on next page)

Table 1
(continued)

Reference/ No. of Studies	No. of Patients (Open/MIS PD)	EBL	Operative Time	POPF/Overall Compilations	LOS	Margins	Nodes	Conclusions
Pędziwiatr et al,[25] 2017	1481/705	Less with MIS PD WMD −190.67 mL P<.0001	Longer with MIS PD WMD 64.09 min P = .002	No significant difference P = .78/P = .12	Shorter with MIS PD WMD −2.24 P = .002	No significant difference P = .77	Similar lymph node harvest P = .25	Although MIS PD takes longer, it may be associated with reduced blood loss, shortened LOS, and comparable rate of perioperative complications.
Chen et al,[26] 2017	2338/1064	Less with MIS PD WMD −0.54 mL P<.01	Longer with MIS PD WMD 99.4 min P<.01	No significant difference P = .25/.10	Shorter with MIS PD WMD −3.49 d P<.01	Lower R1 margins for MIS PD P = .04	Similar lymph node harvest P = .13	MIS PD is technically feasible and safe and is associated with less blood loss, faster postoperative recovery, shorter length of hospitalization, and longer operative time
Zhao et al,[27] 2017	11,483/2052	Less with MIS PD WMD −324.47 P = .0002	Longer with MIS PD WMD 67.37 min P = .002	No significant difference P = .84/NR	Shorter with MIS PD WMD −3.14 d P<.01	Lower R1 margins for MIS PD P<.001	Similar lymph node harvest P = .57	MIS PD can be a reasonable alternative to OPD, but should only be performed at high-volume centers

Abbreviations: EBL, estimated blood loss; LOS, length of stay; MD, mean difference; MIS PD, minimally invasive pancreaticoduodenectomy; POPF, postoperative pancreatic fistula; WMD, weighted mean difference.

Data from Refs.[18–27]

groups throughout the world have described their results and methods of approach to distal lesions of the pancreas. Certainly, laparoscopic left-sided pancreatic resections have more readily been accepted than right-sided pancreaticoduodenectomies because of less extensive dissection and the absences for the need of performing a reconstruction.

Technique

The senior author (H.J.A.) has published and described a "clockwise" technique for left-sided pancreatic resections.[31] The patient is positioned in a modified right lateral decubitus position and secured well to the operative table because the patient's position may need to be adjusted during the case. Reverse Trendelenburg adjustment to the bed allows for gravity retraction that facilitates the dissection and exposure to the spleen and distal pancreas as well as allows for the colon to maximally drop caudally. Two 12-mm and two 5-mm trocars are placed in a semilunar fashion around the body and tail of the pancreas. A 5-step "clockwise" method is used (**Fig. 9**):

The first step focuses on colon mobilization at the splenic flexure. The patient is rotated to the right and into a Trendelenburg position. Lateral attachments of the descending colon are taken down, and this is followed to the splenocolic and gastrocolic ligaments. A window is created at the most lateral portion of the lesser sac, immediately anterior to the distal portion of the tail of the pancreas and immediately medial to the spleen. The window is carried cranially, and the short gastric vessels are ligated and divided fully. Dissection is then carried from left to right progressively dividing the gastrocolic omentum and taking down the attachments to the inferior edge of the pancreas. Depending on the location of the lesion, the inferior mesenteric vein and ligament of Treitz are exposed. The patient is rotated toward the left if required when the dissection needs to be extended more medially toward the neck of the pancreas. Posterior attachments of the stomach to the pancreas are freed. A site is chosen for the division of the pancreas, usually under ultrasound guidance. Next, a window posterior to the pancreas is made separating it from the retroperitoneal attachments.

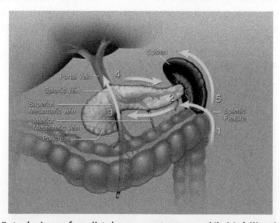

Fig. 9. "Stepwise" technique for distal pancreatectomy. (*1*) Mobilization of the splenic flexure and descending colon. (*2*) Inferior dissection and mobilization of the pancreas and splenic vessels. (*3*) Dissection of the neck of the pancreas. (*4*) Mobilization of the superior portion of the pancreas. (*5*) Spleen mobilization. (*From* Asbun, HJ & Stauffer, JA. Laporascopic approach to distal and subtotal pancreatectomy: a clockwise technique. Springer Science+Business Media, LLC. 2011; 25:2643–9; used with permission of Mayo Foundation for Medical Education and Research, all rights reserved)

Now, focus is targeted at pancreatic and vascular division (splenic artery and vein). The authors use a laparoscopic band-passer to allow for a Penrose drain to be passed around the pancreas proximal to the lesion to allow for retraction off the retroperitoneum. At this point, if splenic preservation is intended, separation of the vessels from the pancreas should be performed. A linear stapler is used in a progressively compressive fashion over several minutes (**Fig. 10**). Tissue staples of at least 4 mm are used with staple-line reinforcement in the authors' practice. The stapler is closed until resistance is felt and held in place for 15 to 30 seconds and then repeated until the stapler is eventually closed completely. Both the vessels and the pancreatic tissue are often included in one stapler load together when including splenectomy.

The pancreas is then retracted and separated further off the retroperitoneum from right to left following a clockwise dissection toward the spleen. Adjacent organs or tissue may be removed en bloc if needed, or the adrenal gland, to obtain an R0 resection.

The principles of R0 resection remain true in this scenario as it does in all attempts of curative resection for cancer. Distal resections may also include local organ resection, including Gerota fascia, transverse mesocolon, splenectomy, adrenalectomy, partial gastrectomy, or colectomy. Again, vascular resection and/or reconstruction may be required.[1]

Outcomes of Minimally Invasive Distal Pancreatectomy

It has been shown in multiple reviews that the laparoscopic approach to distal pancreatectomy is superior to the open distal pancreatectomy (ODP) in several ways. Benefits include transfusion rates and blood loss as well as hospital length of stay. Stauffer and colleagues[32] examined 44 LDP and 28 ODP patients treated for adenocarcinoma of the pancreas at a single institution. Blood loss and transfusion rate were significantly less in the LDP group. Operative time was similar in both groups as was postoperative morbidity, including fistulas, abscess, wound infections, and reoperation. Length of hospital stay was 5.1 days versus 9.4 days favoring LDP ($P = .0001$). The 5-year survival was similar between the 2 groups despite a greater lymph node harvest accomplished in the LDP group (25.9 vs 12.7, $P = .0001$). Nationwide data from the Netherlands further support these findings regarding less blood loss and shorter hospital stay; however, data did show that there was significant selection bias among

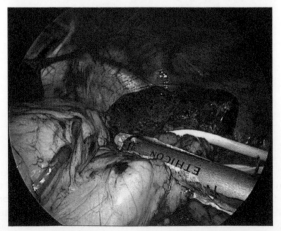

Fig. 10. Sequential compression and stapling for a distal pancreatectomy. A Penrose drain is used to facilitate retraction during the procedure. (*Courtesy of* Ethicon, Inc, Sommerville, NJ.)

surgeons between whom was offered a laparoscopic approach in the treatment of pancreatic cancer.[33] Ricci and colleagues[34] performed a large systematic review of studies comparing LDP to ODP. They identified 5 comparative case control studies, totally 261 patients (30.7% LDP and 69.3% ODP). Again, less blood loss and a shorter hospital stay was significant for the LDP group when compared with the open approach. Overall morbidity, including fistula and leak, reoperation, mortality, and lymph node harvest, was equal between the groups without any effect on overall survival. Consensus is that laparoscopy for distal cancers is at least safe and feasible as an oncologic approach to R0 resection.

The laparoscopic approach to distal pancreatectomy is more technically feasible, but progression to robotic-assisted laparoscopic resection has also been extensively published. Guerrini and colleagues[35] performed a meta-analysis of the data in 2017 looking at 10 studies, including 813 patients. Overall, there was no difference in oncologic outcome, morbidity, or mortality. However, robotic distal pancreatectomy (RDP) was associated with higher rate of splenic preservation (48.9% vs 27%), lower rate of conversion to the open approach (8.2% vs 21.6%), and a shorter hospital stay than the laparoscopic group (7.18 vs 9.08 days). One could argue that both the splenic preservation and the lower rate of conversion to open procedure may be due to ease of the robotic learning curve compared with laparoscopy for some surgeons and may not represent a difference in experienced laparoscopic surgeons, as demonstrated in other series.[32] When comparing with the open approach, cost was higher in the RDP group overall. Many studies, however, show that cost is equivalent between and open and laparoscopic approach due to the shorter hospital stay, but higher operative supply cost for LDP compared with ODP.[36–38]

Regarding oncologic outcomes for LDP versus ODP, no randomized study has been completed to date. The DIPLOMA study, a pan-European propensity score match study for pancreatic adenocarcinoma, sought to examine outcomes for LDP versus ODP.[39] Matched were 1212 patients from 34 centers in 11 countries. Median blood loss and length of stay were lower in the LDP group. Morbidity and mortality were comparable, whereas lymph node retrieval was lower in the LDP group. Median overall survival was similar between LDP versus ODP (28 vs 31 months, $P = .929$) leading to the conclusion that oncologic outcome is, at least, equivalent between techniques. This led to the development of the LEOPARD study protocol for a randomized controlled trial in Europe.[40] This trial seeks to enroll a total of 102 patients in all 17 centers of the Dutch Pancreatic Cancer Group to undergo LDP or ODP with an ERAS-based postsurgical recovery environment. Primary outcomes will look at days to functional recovery, pain control, and hospitalization data. Secondary outcomes include morbidity and mortality, quality of life, and costs. Their data, to date, have been recently presented at the Americas Hepato-Pancreato-Biliary Association 2018 annual meeting showing more favorable results with a minimally invasive surgical approach.[9]

CENTRAL PANCREATIC RESECTION

Minimally invasive central pancreatectomy (CP) is an advanced laparoscopic procedure with select indications. It requires very similar laparoscopic or robotic surgical skills to minimally invasive pancreaticoduodenectomy. CP is indicated in patients with benign or low-grade malignancies in the neck or proximal body of the pancreas. The benefit of CP is sparing parenchyma of the distal pancreas, thus, theoretically reducing the likelihood of postoperative diabetes. However, this benefit must be tempered with a potentially higher rate of postoperative complications compared with minimally invasive distal pancreatectomy.[41] The leak rate after minimally invasive CP is typically higher than that of minimally invasive distal pancreatectomy, because CP results in 2 possible sites for pancreatic leak to occur: proximally, at the transected pancreas, and distally, at the pancreatic anastomosis. Compared with the open approach, the minimally invasive approach to CP was reported to be associated with decreased blood loss, shorter length of hospital stays, faster recovery, and improved quality of life for patients.[42]

Technique

Port number and placement for laparoscopic CP are similar to that of LDP (as described previously) with the exception that the epigastric 5-mm port is placed further to the patient's right, near to the midclavicular line. The operation is begun like LDP with mobilization of the left colon and hepatic flexure. The lesser sac is similarly entered from the patient's left through the gastrocolic omentum. The gastrosplenic ligament and short gastric vessels are divided. The gastrocolic omentum is divided further to the patient's right, exposing the pancreas. The posterior attachments of the stomach to the anterior surface of the pancreas are divided. Next, laparoscopic ultrasound is performed to confirm the location of the underlying lesion as well as to identify the sites of eventual pancreatic transection. Next, a plane is developed between the inferior border of the pancreas and the transverse mesocolon. Depending on the location of the lesion, usually the SMV is identified and retropancreatic tunnel is created between the SMV/PV posteriorly and the neck of the pancreas anteriorly until the superior border of the pancreas is reached. The gland is then encircled with a Penrose drain, taking care to exclude the common hepatic artery and splenic artery. The gland is further separated laterally from the underlying splenic vein distal to the pancreatic pathologic condition. An endoscopic stapler with Peri-Strip reinforcement is then used to transect the pancreas proximal and distal to the pathologic lesion using slow sequential compression as described earlier. At this point, the specimen can be extracted, or this can be done after the reconstruction.

The authors use a pancreaticogastrostomy (PG) or pancreaticojejunostomy to reestablish continuity between the pancreas and gastrointestinal tract. For the

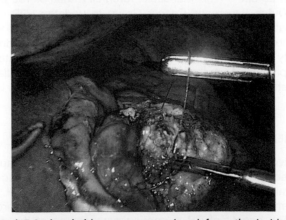

Fig. 11. Interrupted 5-0 absorbable sutures are placed from the inside of the stomach anchoring the cut edge of the pancreas to the cut edge of the posterior wall of the stomach through an anterior gastrostomy during creation of a PG.

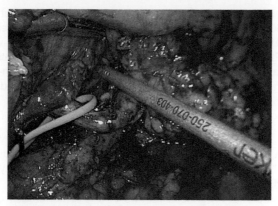

Fig. 12. Posterior gastric view of PG. (Styker Co., Kalamazoo, MI.)

construction of the PG, first, an approximately 5- to 6-cm gastrotomy is made on the anterior surface of the stomach as well as a posterior gastrotomy, approximating the diameter of the gland, which will facilitate passage of the pancreas into the stomach. Interrupted stitches are placed from the inside of the stomach anchoring the cut edge of the pancreas to the cut edge of the posterior wall of the stomach (**Figs. 11** and **12**). The Peri-Strip reinforced staple line on the cut edge of the distal pancreas is excised sharply, and the underlying pancreatic duct is identified. A small pancreatic duct stent is placed, and a ductoplasty is performed using fine interrupted absorbable stitches to marsupialize the often tiny (<3 mm) duct. A seromuscular purse-string stitch is then placed on the outer wall of the posterior stomach surrounding the entering pancreas, creating a seal around the gland. Alternatively, a purse-string suture could be placed initially before opening the posterior wall of the stomach and now tightened at this stage. The anterior gastrotomy is then closed, and a drain is placed posterior to the stomach near the anastomosis. Alternatively, a Roux-en-Y limb of jejunum can be created and a pancreaticojejunostomy can be performed using a technique similar to that of pancreaticoduodenectomy. Drain output and amylase levels are routinely monitored, and drains are removed once appropriate.

SUMMARY

The undertaking of a minimally invasive approach to pancreatic cancer requires expertise, institutional resources, and the willingness and commitment to undergo a learning curve. What is known about laparoscopy in pancreatic adenocarcinoma is that it allows for a shorter hospital stay, less blood loss, less pain, fewer wound complications (early and late), and a quicker return to work and adjuvant therapy. At the very least, oncologic outcomes are equivalent. Furthermore, a minimally invasive approach is safe and feasible. As stated earlier, further controlled studies are needed to assess outcomes as well as cost-benefit given the advantages in laparoscopy previously mentioned. Although many have embraced distal and subtotal pancreatectomy, right-sided resection has a much steeper learning curve and takes the utmost advanced skills in minimally invasive surgery. It is clear that today there is no justification for a surgeon or institution to start embarking into the minimally invasive approach for pancreas resections without appropriate training and implementation. Recent literature further reinforces the need for adequate volume when implementing these techniques. Kutlu and colleagues[43] reviewed the National Cancer Database revealing 4739 patients (4309 OPD and 430 LPD) who had undergone pancreaticoduodenectomy between 2010 and 2011. What was shown was that hospitals with low volume (defined as ≤25 PDs per year) had the highest 30- and 90-day mortality, highest positive margin rate, and lowest lymph node counts. There are many high-volume centers that are practicing this approach on a routine basis and are willing and able to assist in the implementation and training process.

REFERENCES

1. Tempero MA, Malafa MP, Al-Hawary M, et al. Pancreatic adenocarcinoma, version 2.2017, NCCN clinical practice guidelines in oncology. J Natl Compr Canc Netw 2017;15(8):1028–61.
2. Yeo CJ, Cameron JL. Prognostic factors in ductal pancreatic cancer. Langenbecks Arch Surg 1998;383(2):129.
3. Siegel RL, Miller KD, Jemal A. Cancer statistics, 2016. CA Cancer J Clin 2016; 66(1):7–30.
4. Cameron JL, Riall TS, Coleman J, et al. One thousand consecutive pancreaticoduodenectomies. Ann Surg 2006;244(1):10–5.
5. Hyder O, Dodson RM, Nathan H, et al. Influence of patient, physician, and hospital factors on 30-day readmission following pancreatoduodenectomy in the United States. JAMA Surg 2013;148(12):1095.
6. Adam MA, Choudhury K, Dinan MA, et al. Minimally invasive versus open pancreaticoduodenectomy for cancer. Ann Surg 2015;262(2):372–7.
7. Soper NJ, Brunt LM, Dunnegan DL, et al. Laparoscopic distal pancreatectomy in the porcine model. Surg Endosc 1994;8(1):57–61.
8. Stauffer JA, Asbun HJ. Minimally invasive pancreatic surgery. Semin Oncol 2015; 42(1):123–33.
9. De rooij T. Minimally invasive versus open distal pancreatectomy (LEOPARD): multicenter patient-blinded randomized controlled trial. AHPBA 2018. AHPBA 2018 Annual Meeting. Miami, FL, March 9, 2018.
10. Gagner M, Pomp A. Laparoscopic pylorus-preserving pancreatoduodenectomy. Surg Endosc 1994;8(5):408–10.
11. Sosa JA, Bowman HM, Gordon TA, et al. Importance of hospital volume in the overall management of pancreatic cancer. Ann Surg 1998;228(3):429–38.
12. Hogg ME, Besselink MG, Clavien PA, et al. Training in minimally invasive pancreatic resections: a paradigm shift away from 'see one, do one, teach one'. HPB (Oxford) 2017;19(3):234–45.
13. Boggi U, Amorese G, Vistoli F, et al. Laparoscopic pancreaticoduodenectomy: a systematic literature review. Surg Endosc 2014;29(1):9–23.
14. Doula C, Kostakis ID, Damaskos C, et al. Comparison between minimally invasive and open pancreaticoduodenectomy. Surg Laparosc Endosc Percutan Tech 2016;26(1):6–16.
15. Croome KP, Farnell MB, Que FG, et al. Total laparoscopic pancreaticoduodenectomy for pancreatic ductal adenocarcinoma. Ann Surg 2014;260(4):633–40.
16. Stauffer JA, Coppola A, Villacreses D, et al. Laparoscopic versus open pancreaticoduodenectomy for pancreatic adenocarcinoma: long-term results at a single institution. Surg Endosc 2016;31(5):2233–41.
17. Conrad C, Basso V, Passot G, et al. Comparable long-term oncologic outcomes of laparoscopic versus open pancreaticoduodenectomy for adenocarcinoma: a propensity score weighting analysis. Surg Endosc 2017;31(10):3970–8.

18. Correa-Gallego C, Dinkelspiel HE, Sulimanoff I, et al. Minimally-invasive vs open pancreaticoduodenectomy: systematic review and a meta-analysis. J Am Coll Surg 2014;218(1):129–39.

19. Nigri G, Petrucciani N, La Torre M, et al. Duodenopancreatectomy: open or minimally invasive approach? Surgeon 2014;12(4):227–34.

20. Qin H, Qiu J, Zhao Y, et al. Does minimally-invasive pancreaticoduodenectomy have advantages over its open method? a meta-analysis of retrospective studies. PLoS One 2014;9(8):e104274.

21. Lei P, Wei B, Guo W, et al. Minimally invasive surgical approach compared with open pancreaticoduodenectomy: a systematic review and meta-analysis on the feasibility and safety. Surg Laparosc Endosc Percutan Tech 2014;24(4):296–305.

22. de Rooij T, Lu MZ, Steen MW, et al. Minimally invasive versus open pancreatoduodenectomy. Ann Surg 2016;264(2):257–67.

23. Zhang H, Wu X, Zhu F, et al. Systematic review and meta-analysis of minimally invasive versus open approach for pancreaticoduodenectomy. Surg Endosc 2016;30(12):5173–84.

24. Wang S, Shi N, You L, et al. Minimally invasive surgical approach versus open procedure for pancreaticoduodenectomy. Medicine 2017;96:50.

25. Pędziwiatr M, Małczak P, Pisarska M, et al. Minimally invasive versus open pancreatoduodenectomy: a systematic review and meta-analysis. Langenbecks Arch Surg 2017;402(5):841–51.

26. Chen K, Pan Y, Liu XL, et al. Minimally invasive pancreaticoduodenectomy for periampullary disease: a comprehensive review of literature and meta-analysis of outcomes compared with open surgery. BMC Gastroenterol 2017;17(1):120.

27. Zhao Z, Yin Z, Hang Z, et al. A systemic review and an updated meta-analysis: minimally invasive vs open pancreaticoduodenectomy. Sci Rep 2017;7(1):2220.

28. Mesleh MG, Stauffer JA, Bowers SP, et al. Cost analysis of open and laparoscopic pancreaticoduodenectomy: a single institution comparison. Surg Endosc 2013; 27(12):4518–23.

29. Gerber MH, Delitto D, Crippen CJ, et al. Analysis of the cost effectiveness of laparoscopic pancreatoduodenectomy. J Gastrointest Surg 2017;21(9):1404–10.

30. Chen XM, Sun DL, Zhang Y. Laparoscopic versus open pancreaticoduodenectomy combined with uncinated process approach: a comparative study evaluating perioperative outcomes (retrospective cohort study). Int J Surg 2018;51: 170–3.

31. Asbun HJ, Stauffer JA. Laparoscopic approach to distal and subtotal pancreatectomy: a clockwise technique. Surg Endosc 2011;25(8):2643–9.

32. Stauffer JA, Coppola A, Mody K, et al. Laparoscopic versus open distal pancreatectomy for pancreatic adenocarcinoma. World J Surg 2016;40(6):1477–84.

33. de Rooij T, Jilesen AP, Boerma D, et al. A nationwide comparison of laparoscopic and open distal pancreatectomy for benign and malignant disease. J Am Coll Surg 2015;220(3):263–70.e1.

34. Ricci C, Casadei R, Taffurelli G, et al. Laparoscopic versus open distal pancreatectomy for ductal adenocarcinoma: a systematic review and meta-analysis. J Gastrointest Surg 2015;19(4):770–81.

35. Guerrini GP, Lauretta A, Belluco C, et al. Robotic versus laparoscopic distal pancreatectomy: an up-to-date meta-analysis. BMC Surg 2017;17(1):105.

36. Ielpo B, Duran H, Diaz E, et al. Robotic versus laparoscopic distal pancreatectomy: a comparative study of clinical outcomes and costs analysis. Int J Surg 2017;48:300–4.

37. Gurusamy KS, Riviere D, van Laarhoven CJH, et al. Cost-effectiveness of laparoscopic versus open distal pancreatectomy for pancreatic cancer. Plos One 2017; 12(12):e0189631.
38. Ricci C, Casadei R, Taffurelli G, et al. Laparoscopic distal pancreatectomy in benign or premalignant pancreatic lesions: is it really more cost-effective than open approach? J Gastrointest Surg 2015;19(8):1415–24.
39. van Hilst J, de Rooij T, Klompmaker S, et al. Minimally invasive versus open distal pancreatectomy for ductal adenocarcinoma (DIPLOMA): a pan-european propensity score matched study. Ann Surg 2017;1. https://doi.org/10.1097/sla.0000000000002561.
40. de Rooij T, van Hilst J, Vogel JA, et al. Minimally invasive versus open distal pancreatectomy (LEOPARD): study protocol for a randomized controlled trial. Trials 2017;18(1):166.
41. Song KB, Kim SC, Park KM, et al. Laparoscopic central pancreatectomy for benign or low-grade malignant lesions in the pancreatic neck and proximal body. Surg Endosc 2014;29(4):937–46.
42. Zhang RC, Zhang B, Mou YP, et al. Comparison of clinical outcomes and quality of life between laparoscopic and open central pancreatectomy with pancreaticojejunostomy. Surg Endosc 2017;31(11):4756–63.
43. Kutlu OC, Lee JE, Katz MH, et al. Open pancreaticoduodenectomy case volume predicts outcome of laparoscopic approach. Ann Surg 2018;267(3):552–60.

Minimally Invasive Small Bowel Cancer Surgery

Ioana Baiu, MD, MPH[a], Brendan C. Visser, MD[b],*

KEYWORDS

- Small bowel cancer • Small bowel GIST • Small bowel adenocarcinoma
- Small bowel lymphoma • Small bowel neuroendocrine tumor • Carcinoid
- Minimally invasive surgery • Laparoscopic surgery

KEY POINTS

- Small bowel cancers are very rare, and there are limited data regarding surgical techniques.
- Minimally invasive approaches for small bowel tumors are safe and feasible.
- Although there are very limited data, the risk of postoperative complications appears to favor laparoscopic techniques without compromising surgical outcomes.

INTRODUCTION

Although the small intestine represents 75% of the length and 90% of the functional absorptive capacity of the gastrointestinal tract, small bowel tumors account for only 2% of the gastrointestinal malignancies.[1] In 2018, the American Cancer Society estimates 1,735,350 expected new diagnoses of cancer, of which 319,160 of the digestive system, and only 10,470 primarily of the small intestine.[1] Nevertheless, the incidence of small bowel malignancies has increased dramatically over the past 30 years, partly due to improved imaging techniques and the increased prevalence of immunocompromised patients. Notably, the United States has the highest age-adjusted incidence of this type of cancer in the world.[2] The relative inaccessibility of the small intestine endoscopically contributes to delays in diagnosis. Indeed, there have been no major improvements in outcomes and long-term survival in small bowel malignancies in the past 20 years, and the treatment recommendations have remained largely unchanged.[3] The primary treatment of these malignancies is surgical resection.

Disclosure Statement: The authors have no extramural funding or conflicts of interest to disclose.
^a Department of Surgery, Stanford University School of Medicine, 300 Pasteur Drive, H3561, Stanford, CA 94305, USA; ^b Department of Surgery, Stanford University School of Medicine, 300 Pasteur Drive, H3680, Stanford, CA 94305, USA
* Corresponding author.
E-mail address: bvisser@stanford.edu

surgonc.theclinics.com

As technology has evolved, minimally invasive techniques have allowed resection of small bowel tumors with reduced morbidity without compromising outcomes.[4]

MALIGNANT TUMORS OF THE SMALL BOWEL

A 2007 single-institution review of 1260 small bowel tumors found 33% to be carcinoid, 30% adenocarcinoma, 16% lymphoma, 7% gastrointestinal stromal tumor (GIST), and 13% of other type (melanoma, breast, colon, ovary, uterus, stomach metastases).[5]

Neuroendocrine Tumors of the Small Intestine

Small bowel neuroendocrine tumors (NETs) (traditionally termed carcinoid tumors) are malignant NETs that arise in the crypts of Lieberkühn. The incidence of small bowel NETs has increased fourfold in recent decades, becoming the most common malignant neoplasm of the small intestine.[3] This trend parallels the increased incidence of all gastrointestinal NETs, which are now the second-most common malignancy of the gastrointestinal tract after colorectal cancer.[6] Most NETs occur in the ileum, specifically in the distal 60 cm of the ileum.[5,7] Up to one-third of patients present with multiple tumors, and regional lymph node metastases occur 60% of the time.[8] Tumors larger than 1 cm with invasion of the muscularis propria have a higher likelihood of metastasis.[9] Most patients are asymptomatic; liver or retroperitoneal metastases may lead to systemic symptoms (carcinoid syndrome) related to secretory products, such as serotonin, histamine, prostaglandins.

Surgical resection of the small bowel NETs is often indicated across the spectrum of disease, from incidentally found tumors to those patients with metastases at diagnosis.[10,11] In the case of metastatic disease, surgical resection of the primary tumor will likely not impact the systemic symptoms, but there may be a survival benefit because unresected local disease can result in debilitating bowel obstruction late in the course of the disease (due to either luminal obstruction tumor or cicatrization and tethering of the small bowel by mesenteric nodes). Although no randomized controlled trials exist regarding small bowel NET surgery, laparoscopic resection has been found to be safe and feasible.[12] Because of the high tendency of NETs to metastasize to regional lymph nodes, preoperative imaging is essential in determining if a minimally invasive approach is practical. Contrast-enhanced multiphasic computed tomography (CT) remains the most useful modality for operative planning, although Gallium-68 DOTATATE PET-CT now plays an essential role in identifying a small occult primary and identifying whether mesenteric nodes are involved.[13] There are several important clinical and technical considerations in planning resection of small bowel NETs. Modest-sized ileal and jejunal tumors with limited nodal involvement are the best candidates for a minimally invasive approach. If the involved nodes have descended to the root of the mesentery, resection of a larger segment of small bowel and/or dissection right onto the superior mesenteric artery or superior mesenteric vein may be required, which makes a laparoscopic approach extremely challenging and may not be safe. Nodes left behind at the root of the mesentery may contribute to late morbidity (obstruction), so involved nodes should be resected whenever feasible (and adequate length of bowel left behind). A subset of patients will present with clinically visible nodes but without an overt primary. These patients will require close inspection and palpation of the small bowel to identify the primary (including the possibility of multifocality). In these cases, laparoscopy may be limiting, as it does not provide the same tactile feedback of an open resection,[8] although a hand-assisted approach or a very small incision to briefly exteriorize and "run the bowel" may still allow a laparoscopic-assisted resection. Distal NETs, such as those that occur in the terminal ileum, typically require a laparoscopic right hemicolectomy to adequately harvest the ileocolic lymph nodes, which has been showed to be feasible and safe in the colorectal literature. Finally, there are isolated case reports of laparoscopic or robotic resection of duodenal NETs, typically small (1 cm or smaller) tumors away from the ampulla permitting a local, full-thickness excision.[8,14] Finally, in patients with metastatic small bowel NET who are undergoing laparoscopic resection of the primary, consideration should be made to concomitant laparoscopic cholecystectomy, because long-term treatment with somatostatin receptor inhibitors is well-known to result in gallstone formation, which can lead to morbidity later in the course of the disease.[15]

Adenocarcinoma

Adenocarcinoma is the second-most common tumor of the small bowel. Although it can arise throughout the entire small intestine, 56% of tumors are located in the duodenum.[3] Similar to the large bowel, adenomatous polyps can have malignant degeneration leading to the development of adenocarcinoma. One of the main risk factors for the development of small intestinal adenocarcinoma is Crohn disease, both due to chronic inflammation as well as immunosuppressive treatments.[16,17] Surgical resection is the mainstay of treatment and can be curative in 40% to 65% of cases.[17–20] Tumors located in the second portion of the duodenum require a pancreaticoduodenectomy. Those in the first, third, and fourth portions can be removed using segmental resection. The importance of lymphadenectomy in adenocarcinoma is important, as greater lymph node retrieval for duodenal adenocarcinoma may be independently associated with improved survival.[21,22] Studies have shown that adequate staging requires a minimum of 5 lymph nodes for duodenal adenocarcinoma, and 9 lymph nodes for jejunoileal adenocarcinoma.[21] Although more radical resection (pancreaticoduodenectomy) offers a significantly greater lymph node retrieval, segmental resection of the tumor has been shown to have an equal survival benefit.[23] Both minimally invasive pancreaticoduodenectomy and segmental resection for small bowel adenocarcinoma are feasible in select cases as long as oncologic principles of margin-negative resection and adequate lymphadenectomy are followed.

Lymphoma

The small intestine is the most frequent extranodal site for non-Hodgkin lymphoma.[24] The small intestine contains lymphoid tissue, making it prone to malignant transformation into lymphoma. As such, 65% of gastrointestinal lymphomas are found in the terminal ileum, where the greatest concentration of lymphoid tissue exists; 25% in the jejunum, and 10% in the duodenum.[25] Lymphoma in the small bowel most commonly presents with intussusception, obstruction, or bleeding.[26] Although surgical resection of gastric lymphomas has not been shown to be beneficial,[27,28] the role of surgery in small bowel lymphoma is not as clearly elucidated. Surgery has been used primarily in patients with bulky disease, tumor-related complications such as bowel-perforation or intestinal obstruction, or for diagnostic purposes with the goal of obtaining adequate tissue for pathology to subtype the lymphoma for treatment planning.[29] Up to one-third of patients may present with multifocal lymphoma; another third of cases present with tumors in the ileocecal valve.[29] Bulky or multifocal disease and the presence of complications (obstruction or perforation with peritonitis) may limit a minimally invasive approach. Many surgeons choose to complete the small bowel anastomosis via an extracorporeal approach using a hand-assisted port or similar at the site of specimen extraction.[30]

Gastrointestinal Stromal Tumor

GISTs are the most common sarcomas of the gastrointestinal tract and are most commonly found in the stomach and small intestine. GISTs arise from the interstitial cells of Cajal and occur in patients older than 50 in the stomach (60%), jejunum and ileum (30%), duodenum (5%), colon and appendix (1%), and esophagus (>1%).[31,32] Compared with gastric tumors, small bowel GISTs have a worse prognosis and have a higher risk of metastases.[32] Despite advancements in molecular targeted therapies, surgery is the only curative option.[33,34] Lymph node metastasis is quite rare in gastric tumors (5%), but more common in small bowel GISTs (18%).[35] Large data analyses do show a negative impact in survival with lymph node involvement.[35] Nevertheless, the current surgical principles require an R0 resection with no systemic lymph node dissection, unless the nodes are clinically enlarged.[36] Minimally invasive approaches to gastric GISTs have been widely described and accepted,[37–39] and multiple studies have described the feasibility and safety of laparoscopic small bowel resections.[31,37,40–42] As stromal tumors, GISTs are highly vascular, and rupture has been associated with life-threatening bleeding as well as spread of the tumor to the abdominal cavity. The European Society for Medical Oncology 2004 consensus notes that GISTs should be resected through a minimally invasive approach only if they are 2 cm or smaller, as there is a high risk for capsular rupture using laparoscopic forceps. However, with improved techniques, tumors as large as 10 cm can be resected laparoscopically with minimal manipulation on the tissue.[39,43] Overall, the literature suggests that minimally invasive approaches are often appropriate for small bowel GISTs that are modest in size (eg, <5 cm) and that are not too soft or fragile.[38,44] The technical key is to avoid direct manipulation of the tumor itself, instead handling the adjacent small bowel and mesentery. The mesentery can be divided reasonably close to the tumor itself. Once the involved segment of bowel and tumor is resected, it should be carefully bagged before extraction given the risk of spillage and resultant "GISTosis."

BENIGN TUMORS OF THE SMALL BOWEL

Adenomas, Brunneromas, lipomas, hemangiomas, hamartomas, GISTs, and leiomyomas are all benign tumors that can be found in the small intestine. The main indication for operative resection of these neoplasms is symptom management (obstruction, intussusception, hemorrhage) or to rule out malignancy. The treatment of benign small intestinal tumors depends on the size, location, and potential for malignancy. Treatment options include endoscopic snare excision, minimally invasive wedge or partial resections, and radical duodenectomy or pancreaticoduodenectomy, although no clear guidelines exist. Adenomas and Brunneromas can typically be resected endoscopically. Adenomas tend to grow in the second portion of the duodenum and are less common in the distal intestine.[45] Just as with colonic polyps that have malignant degeneration, up to 30% of periampullary adenomas and villous adenomas of the small bowel have malignant potential.[46] Radical resections are generally indicated only when malignant growth is detected on pathology. Leiomyomas occur in the jejunum but cannot be clinically distinguished from leiomyosarcoma and therefore warrant resection. Hamartomas are typically found in the jejunum and ileum and have a low malignant potential. Last, lipomas should be excised only when causing symptoms such as bowel obstruction.

As the use of routine esophagoduodenoscopy (EGD) has increased, so has the early detection of benign or premalignant tumors of the duodenum. Although 0.3% to 4.6% of routine EGDs will detect a benign tumor, the surgical management of these neoplasms is still under debate. Endoscopic resection has been established as being successful in proximal lesions such as periampullary and duodenal adenomas,[13,47–52] but may be associated with incomplete resection and high recurrence rate.[53,54] Furthermore, endoscopic resection is typically recommended for pedunculated, superficial lesions smaller than 1 cm in easy to reach locations, and without submucosal invasion. In larger lesions and/or those that have submucosal involvement, surgical resection is the preferred treatment. Hand-assisted laparoscopic duodenal mobilization and open local excision technique for benign duodenal neoplasms has been described as a safe, effective, and faster alternative when a pure laparoscopic approach would be technically too difficult.[55]

SURGICAL CONSIDERATIONS BASED ON ANATOMIC LOCATION
Duodenum

Duodenal surgery involves complex anatomic relationships, and minimally invasive techniques pose challenges for adequate dissection. Tumors located in D1 and D4 are amenable to limited duodenal resection. Laparoscopically, this is easier achieved with the patient in split-leg position and the surgeon operating from between the legs. This allows for an adequate angle when dissecting the duodenum and regional lymph nodes. A Billroth II reconstruction is typically used for D1 resections, and the ease of a single anastomosis makes it amenable to minimally invasive approaches. This has not only proven durability but also allows for retrograde access to the remaining duodenum via esophagogastroduodenoscopy. D2 and periampullary D3 tumors require pancreaticoduodenectomy and the reconstruction of the hepatic and pancreatic anastomoses to the jejunum. Most D2 and D3 resections continue to be performed via the open approach.[56] When performed via an open technique, resection of D3 and D4 is often achieved using variations on the Cattell-Braasch technique.[57] In contrast, minimally invasive (laparoscopic or robotic) D3 and D4 resections are achieved working under the mesentery from the midline. The patient is placed in the lithotomy, allowing the surgeon to work from between the legs. The transverse colon is retracted cephalad. After mobilizing the bowel at the ligament of Treitz, the proximal jejunum is divided just distal to that point and the mesentery of this segment of jejunum and the forth portion of the duodenum is divided with a vessel sealing device. The avascular area of the peritoneum of the transverse mesocolon in then incised on the right side of the root of the mesentery to allow the mobilized segment of bowel to be passed under the root of the mesentery and delivered on the right side. Placement of a balloon catheter via the cystic duct (requiring cholecystectomy) into the duodenum allows identification and protection of the ampulla. The duodenum is then divided just distal to the ampulla with an endoscopic linear stapler and a side-to-side duodenojejunostomy is performed in the lateral wall opposite the ampulla.[58]

Small Bowel

Small bowel tumors of the jejunum and ileum may pose a challenge laparoscopically when an extensive lymphadenectomy and resection of the mesentery is required. Although laparoscopy is often helpful in running the bowel and visualizing key anatomic structures, it poses technical obstacles with extensive resections. Limited small bowel resections can be achieved via minimally invasive techniques and anastomoses can be constructed laparoscopically, although much of the literature describes an extracorporeal anastomosis because of the relative ease of exteriorizing the ends for a quick reconstruction through the incision required for specimen extraction.

Terminal Ileum

Tumors located in the terminal ileum pose a challenge because of their lymph node drainage. As such, small bowel tumors located in the distal and terminal ileum and that require lymphadenectomy will most likely require a right hemicolectomy. There is a rich literature about the safety and feasibility of laparoscopic colon resections with primary anastomosis, often done via a hand-assisted port.

SURGICAL OUTCOMES

There are several studies that have compared open with laparoscopic techniques for small bowel malignancies. Most of them analyzed GIST resection but the results can be generalized to other small bowel tumors. A retrospective study looked at 12 consecutive patients undergoing surgical resection of duodenal tumors and compared laparoscopic with open. The patients who underwent laparoscopic resection had statistically higher preoperative risks, such increased body mass index, hypertension, diabetes, and gastroesophageal reflux disease. The minimally invasive technique involved extracorporeal anastomosis in 42% of patients and wedge resection of the affected duodenum in 58%. Although the hospital length of stay, and the 30-day and 90-day mortality were similar between the open and minimally invasive groups, the latter had fewer complications, such as ventral hernias and wound infections. There were 2 patients in the laparoscopic group who had positive margins, but no further surgical interventions were necessary and there were no recurrences at a short 12-month follow-up.

Perhaps the largest multi-institutional retrospective review of minimally invasive surgical approaches to benign and premalignant duodenal tumors included 26 patients who underwent robotic duodenal resection.[58] The procedures included ampullectomy, transduodenal excision of mass partial duodenal resection with excision of mass, segmental duodenal resection, or sleeve duodenectomy. The rate of complications at 30 and 90 days was calculated using the Clavien-Dindo classification.[59] Whereas laparoscopy presented some technical challenges for reconstructing the ampulla and the duodenum, the investigators argue that robotic surgery allows for a more versatile and yet safe approach to completing the entire operation in a minimally invasive fashion. There were no conversions to open approach among these 26 patients and the blood loss was minimal. The Clavien-Dindo classification revealed that 50% of patients had no complications, 35% had minor events, and 15% had major events requiring reoperation, interventional radiology drainage, or intensive care unit management. The investigators did not include a control group to compare the complication rates within this multi-institutional analysis. The existing literature points to complications as high as 50% in in pancreaticoduodenectomy compared with 33% in ampullectomy,[60] as well as in open resection for nonampullary neoplasms compared with ampullectomy.[61]

The largest meta-analysis was published in 2017 and analyzed 6 comparative studies, including a total of 391 patients from East Asia. The meta-analysis points to statistically significant benefits of minimally invasive (170 patients, 43.5%) over open approaches (221 patients, 56.5%). Specifically, laparoscopic resection provides a shorter operation time, less intraoperative blood loss, earlier time to flatus and time to restart oral intake, shorter hospital stay, and a decrease in overall complications. They also conclude that there was no statistically significant difference in tumor recurrence and long-term survival between the 2 groups.

Another large meta-analysis reviewed duodenal GIST resection and included 189 patients treated with limited resection (LR) and 105 via open pancreaticoduodenectomy.[62]

The choice of operation was contingent on tumor size, location, relation to the ampulla of Vater, invasion, and patient's overall fitness. Although the investigators note that LR can be achieved laparoscopically, there is no distinction or subanalysis in the study between the minimally invasive and open approaches.

A small retrospective study compared all small bowel tumor resections from 1998 to 2005 and included 9 patients treated with laparoscopy versus 11 patients with open resection.[63] Fifteen of these patients were diagnosed with GIST, with the other 5 being vascular ectasia, schwannoma, inflammatory polyp, and lymphoma. The minimally invasive approach was used if there was no evidence of dissemination of the tumor at the time of surgery. Nearly half of the patients who underwent laparoscopy had had a prior open abdominal surgery. Consistent with other studies, the minimally invasive group had significantly less blood loss, less use of pain medications, shorter time to oral intake, and shorter length of stay. Although the rate of complications was not shown to be statistically significant, 2 patients in the laparoscopy group required readmission and laparotomy for intestinal obstruction. Similarly, 3 patients in the open group were readmitted for wound infections. Yet another group from China reviewed 90 consecutive patients who underwent small bowel stromal tumor resections and compared hand-assisted laparoscopy with open technique.[40] The former approach included intra-abdominal inspection and dissection laparoscopically, with extracorporeal resection and primary anastomosis. Out of the 85 patients without metastases who underwent a primary resection, 38 underwent hand-assisted laparoscopy and 47 open resections. The preoperative criteria for attempting a minimally invasive approach was tumor size smaller than 5 cm. Although the outcomes and complications appear to be similar to prior studies, the investigators also compared medical and surgical costs of each approach and concluded that overall minimally invasive technique was overall cheaper.

Long-term outcomes for small bowel GIST treated with minimally invasive versus open techniques have been shown to be overall equivalent in all of the previously mentioned studies during the follow-up duration. One retrospective study analyzed perioperative outcomes and long-term relapse-free survival in 80 patients who underwent laparoscopy-assisted resection (LAR) versus open resection (OPEN).[41] As predicted, time to oral intake and postoperative hospital duration was significantly shorter in the LAR group. The complication rates were defined using the Clavien-Dindo scale; there was no difference in grade I and V complications, but the OPEN approach had statistically significantly higher risks of grade II, III, and IV complications. The 5-year relapse-free survival was identical in both groups.

DISCUSSION

Given the low incidence of small bowel malignancies, most published work to date consists of case reports or retrospective studies aiming at proving safety and efficacy of minimally invasive approaches to small bowel cancer resections.[64–75] Few studies have focused on the superiority of laparoscopic techniques compared with open approaches, but the data are quite limited by numbers and the study design. As minimally invasive approaches to bowel surgery are undergoing a critical appraisal, the focus remains on benign conditions, such as inflammatory bowel disease, small bowel obstruction secondary to adhesions, or large bowel malignancies.[76–78] To date, there have been no randomized controlled trials that allow for an objective comparison between minimally invasive and open approaches to similar tumors of the small bowel. Despite the severe limitations of existing data, there appear to be benefits in postoperative pain control, duration of hospital stay, and complication rate with laparoscopic techniques without compromising safety, duration of operation, and risk of recurrence in select patients.

REFERENCES

1. Siegel RL, Miller KD, Jemal A. Cancer statistics 2018. CA Cancer J Clin 2018; 68(1):7–30.
2. Haselkorn T, Whittemore AS, Lilienfeld DE. Incidence of small bowel cancer in the United States and worldwide: geographic, temporal, and racial differences. Cancer Causes Control 2005;16(7):781.
3. Bilimoria KY, Bentrem DJ, Wayne JD, et al. Small bowel cancer in the United States: changes in epidemiology, treatment, and survival over the last 20 years. Ann Surg 2009;249(1):63.
4. Jimenez Rodriguez RM, Segura-Sampedro JJ, Flores-Cortés M, et al. Laparoscopic approach in gastrointestinal emergencies. World J Gastroenterol 2016; 22(9):2701–10.
5. Hatzaras I, Palesty JA, Abir F, et al. Small-bowel tumors: epidemoiologic and clinical characteristics of 1260 cases from the Connecticut tumor registry. Arch Surg 2007;142(3):229–35.
6. Yao JC, Hassan M, Phan A, et al. One hundred years after "carcinoid": epidemiology of and prognostic factors for neuroendocrine tumors in 35,825 cases in the United States. J Clin Oncol 2008;26(18):3063–72.
7. Strosberg J. Neuroendocrine tumours of the small intestine. Best Pract Res Clin Gastroenterol 2012;26(6):755–73.
8. Xavier S, Rosa B, Cotter J. Small bowel neuroendocrine tumors: from pathophysiology to clinical approach. World J Gastrointest Pathophysiol 2016;7(1):117–24.
9. Shamiyeh A, Gabriel M. Laparoscopic resection of gastrointestinal neuroendocrine tumors with special contribution of radionuclide imaging. World J Gastroenterol 2014;20:15608–15.
10. Srirajaskanthan R, Ahmed A, Prachialias A, et al. ENETS TNM staging predicts prognosis in small bowel neuroendocrine tumours. ISRN Oncol 2013;2013: 420795.
11. Akerström G, Hellman P, Hessman O, et al. Management of midgut carcinoids. J Surg Oncol 2005;89(3):161–9.
12. Bucher P, Gervaz P, Ris F, et al. Laparoscopic versus open resection for appendix carcinoid. Surg Endosc 2006;20(6):967–70.
13. Alonso O, Rodríguez-Taroco M, Savio E, et al. (68)Ga-DOTATATE PET/CT in the evaluation of patients with neuroendocrine metastatic carcinoma of unknown origin. Ann Nucl Med 2014;28(7):638–45.
14. Abe N, Takeuchi H, Shibuya M, et al. Successful treatment of duodenal carcinoid tumor by laparoscopy-assisted endoscopic full-thickness resection with lymphadenectomy. Asian J Endosc Surg 2012;5(2):81–5.
15. Roti E, Minelli R, Gardini E, et al. Chronic treatment with a long-acting somatostatin analogue in a patient with intestinal carcinoid tumor: occurrence of cholelithiasis. J Endocrinol Invest 1990;13(1):69–72.
16. Lashner BA. Risk factors for small bowel cancer in Crohn's disease. Dig Dis Sci 1992;37(8):1179–84.
17. Neugut AI, Marvin MR, Rella VA, et al. An overview of adenocarcinoma of the small intestine. Oncology (Williston Park) 1997;11(4):529–36.

18. Bauer RL, Palmer ML, Bauer AM, et al. Adenocarcinoma of the small intestine: 21-year review of diagnosis, treatment, and prognosis. Ann Surg Oncol 1994;1(2): 183–8.

19. Neugut AI, Marvin MR, Chabot JA. Surgical treatment: evidence-based and problem-oriented. Adenocarcinoma of the small bowel. Munich (Germany): Zuckschwerdt; 2001.

20. Agrawal S, McCarron EC, Gibbs JF, et al. Surgical management and outcome in primary adenocarcinoma of the small bowel. Ann Surg Oncol 2007;14(8):2263–9.

21. Tran TB, Qadan M, Dua MM, et al. Prognostic relevance of lymph node ratio and total lymph node count for small bowel adenocarcinoma. Surgery 2015;158(2): 486–93.

22. Overman MJ, Hu CY, Wolff RA, et al. Prognostic value of lymph node evaluation in small bowel adenocarcinoma: analysis of the Surveillance, Epidemiology, and End Results database. Cancer 2010;116(23):5374–82.

23. Cloyd JM, Norton JA, Visser BC, et al. Does the extent of resection impact survival for duodenal adenocarcinoma? Analysis of 1,611 cases. Ann Surg Oncol 2015;22:573–80.

24. d'Amore F, Brincker H, Grønbaek K, et al. Non-Hodgkin's lymphoma of the gastrointestinal tract: a population-based analysis of incidence, geographic distribution, clinicopathologic presentation features, and prognosis. Danish Lymphoma Study Group. J Clin Oncol 1994;12(8):1673–84.

25. Schottenfeld D, Beebe-Dimmer JL, Vigneau FD. The epidemiology and pathogenesis of neoplasia in the small intestine. Ann Epidemiol 2009;19(1):58–69.

26. Matsushita M, Hajiro K, Kajiyama T, et al. Malignant lymphoma in the ileocecal region causing intussusception. J Gastroenterol 1994;29(2):203–7.

27. Avilés A, Nambo MJ, Neri N, et al. The role of surgery in primary gastric lymphoma. Results of a controlled clinical trial. Ann Surg 2004;240(1):44–50.

28. Koch P, del Valle F, Berdel WE, et al, German Multicenter Study Group. Primary gastrointestinal non-Hodgkin's lymphoma: II. Combined surgical and conservative or conservative management only in localized gastric lymphoma—results of the prospective German Multicenter Study GIT NHL 01/92. J Clin Oncol 2001;19(18):3874–83.

29. Hong YW, Kuo IM, Liu YY, et al. The role of surgical management in primary small bowel lymphoma: a single-center experience. Eur J Surg Oncol 2017;43(10): 1886–93.

30. Ishibashi Y, Yamamoto S, Yamada Y, et al. Laparoscopic resection for malignant lymphoma of the ileum causing ileocecal intussusception. Surg Laparosc Endosc Percutan Tech 2007;17(5):444–6.

31. Lai ECH, Lau SHY, Lau WY. Current management of gastrointestinal stromal tumors—a comprehensive review. Int J Surg 2012;10(7):334–40.

32. Miettinen M, Lasota J. Gastrointestinal stromal tumors: pathology and prognosis at different sites. Semin Diagn Pathol 2006;23:70–83.

33. Grover S, Ashley SW, Raut CP. Small intestine gastrointestinal stromal tumors. Curr Opin Gastroenterol 2012;28(2):113–23.

34. Demetri GD, von Mehren M, Antonescu CR, et al. NCCN Task Force report: update on the management of patients with gastrointestinal stromal tumors. J Natl Compr Canc Netw 2010;8(2):1–41.

35. Güller U, Tarantino I, Cerny T, et al. Population-based SEER trend analysis of overall and cancer-specific survival in 5138 patients with gastrointestinal stromal tumor. BMC Cancer 2015;15:557.

36. Kong S, Yang H. Surgical treatment of gastric gastrointestinal stromal tumor. J Gastric Cancer 2013;13(1):3–18.

37. Fisher SB, Kim SC, Kooby DA, et al. Gastrointestinal stromal tumors: a single institution experience of 176 surgical patients. Am Surg 2013;79(7):657–65.

38. Otani Y, Furukawa T, Yoshida M, et al. Operative indications for relatively small (2-5 cm) gastrointestinal stromal tumor of the stomach based on analysis of 60 operated cases. Surgery 2006;139(4):484–92.

39. Karakousis GC, Singer S, Zheng J, et al. Laparoscopic versus open gastric resections for primary gastrointestinal stromal tumors (GISTs): a size-matched comparison. Ann Surg Oncol 2011;18(6):1599–605.

40. Cai W, Wang ZT, Wu L, et al. Laparoscopically assisted resections of small bowel stromal tumors are safe and effective. J Dig Dis 2011;12(6):443–7.

41. Wan P, Li C, Yan M, et al. Laparoscopy-assisted versus open surgery for gastrointestinal stromal tumors of jejunum and ileum: perioperative outcomes and long-term follow-up experience. Am Surg 2012;78(12):1399–404.

42. Pitiakoudis M, Zezos P, Courcoutsakis N, et al. Is laparoscopic resection the appropriate management of a jejunal gastrointestinal stromal tumor (GIST)? Report of a case. Surg Laparosc Endosc Percutan Tech 2010;20(5):160–3.

43. Anania G, Dellachiesa L, Fabbri N, et al. Totally laparoscopic resection of a very large gastric GIST. G Chir 2013;34(7–8):227–30.

44. Ryu KJ, Jung SR, Choi JS, et al. Laparoscopic resection of small gastric submucosal tumors. Surg Endosc 2011;25(1):271–7.

45. Greenfield LJ, Mulholland MW, Oldham KT, et al. Greenfield's surgery: scientific principles and practice. 5th edition. Philadelphia: Lippincott Williams and Wilkins; 2006.

46. Sellner F. Investigations on the significance of the adenoma-carcinoma sequence in the small bowel. Cancer 1990;66(4):702–15.

47. Standards of Practice Committee, Adler DG, Qureshi W, et al. The role of endoscopy in ampullary and duodenal adenomas. Gastrointest Endosc 2006;64(6):849–54.

48. Jung JH, Choi KD, Ahn JY, et al. Endoscopic submucosal dissection for sessile, nonampullary duodenal adenomas. Endoscopy 2013;45(2):133–5.

49. Jung MK, Cho CM, Park SY, et al. Endoscopic resection of ampullary neoplasms: a single-center experience. Surg Endosc 2009;23(11):2568–74.

50. Abbass R, Rigaux J, Al-Kawas FH. Nonampullary duodenal polyps: characteristics and endoscopic management. Gastrointest Endosc 2010;71(4):754–9.

51. Patel R, Varadarajulu S, Wilcox CM. Endoscopic ampullectomy: techniques and outcomes. J Clin Gastroenterol 2012;46(1):8–15.

52. Min YW, Min BH, Kim ER, et al. Efficacy and safety of endoscopic treatment for nonampullary sporadic duodenal adenomas. Dig Dis Sci 2013;58(10):2926–32.

53. Tsujimoto H, Ichikura T, Nagao S, et al. Minimally invasive surgery for resection of duodenal carcinoid tumors: endoscopic full-thickness resection under laparoscopic observation. Surg Endosc 2010;24:471–5.

54. Basford PJ, Bhandari P. Endoscopic management of nonampullary duodenal polyps. Therap Adv Gastroenterol 2012;5:127–38.

55. Poultsides GA, Pappou EP, Bloom GP, et al. Hybrid resection of duodenal tumors. J Laparoendosc Adv Surg Tech A 2011;21(7):603–8.

56. Cameron J. Current surgical therapy. 12th edition. Philadelphia (PA): Elsevier Health Sciences; 2016.

57. García-Molina FJ, Mateo-Vallejo F, Franco-Osorio Jde D, et al. Surgical approach for tumours of the third and fourth part of the duodenum. Distal pancreas-sparing duodenectomy. Int J Surg 2015;18:143–8.
58. Downs-Canner S, Van der Vliet WJ, Thoolen SJ, et al. Robotic surgery for benign duodenal tumors. J Gastrointest Surg 2015;19(2):306–12.
59. Dindo D, Demartines N, Clavien PA. Classification of surgical complications: a new proposal with evaluation in a cohort of 6336 patients and results of a survey. Ann Surg 2004;240(2):205–13.
60. Winter JM, Cameron JL, Olino K, et al. Clinicopathologic analysis of ampullary neoplasms in 450 patients: implications for surgical strategy and long-term prognosis. J Gastrointest Surg 2010;14(2):379–87.
61. Kemp CD, Russell RT, Sharp KW. Resection of benign duodenal neoplasms. Am Surg 2007;73(11):1086–91.
62. Chok AY, Koh YX, Ow MY, et al. A systematic review and meta-analysis comparing pancreaticoduodenectomy versus limited resection for duodenal gastrointestinal stromal tumors. Ann Surg Oncol 2014;21(11):3429–38.
63. Tsui DK, Tang CN, Ha JP, et al. Laparoscopic approach for small bowel tumors. Surg Laparosc Endosc Percutan Tech 2008;18(6):556–60.
64. Bowers SP, Smith CD. Laparoscopic resection of posterior duodenal bulb carcinoid tumor. Am Surg 2003;69(9):792–5.
65. Blanc P, Porcheron J, Pages A, et al. Laparoscopic excision of a duodenal neuroendocrine tumor. Ann Chir 2000;125(2):176–8.
66. Van de Walle P, Dillemans B, Vandelanotte M, et al. The laparoscopic resection of a benign stromal tumour of the duodenum. Acta Chir Belg 1997;97(3):127–9.
67. Toyonaga T, Nakamura K, Araki Y, et al. Laparoscopic treatment of duodenal carcinoid tumor. Wedge resection of the duodenal bulb under endoscopic control. Surg Endosc 1998;12(8):1085–7.
68. Adell-Carceller R, Salvador-Sanchis JL, Navarro-Navarro J, et al. Laparoscopically treated duodenal hamartoma of Brunner's glands. Surg Laparosc Endosc 1997;7(4):298–300.
69. Baladas HG, Borody TJ, Smith GS, et al. Laparoscopic excision of a Brunner's gland hamartoma of the duodenum. Surg Endosc 2002;16(11):1636.
70. Shiraishi N, Yasuda K, Bandoh T, et al. Laparoscopic resection for ectopic gastric mucosa of the duodenum: report of a case. Surg Today 1999;29(4):351–3.
71. Cheah WK, Lenzi JE, Chong S, et al. Laparoscopic excision of duodenal tumors. Surg Endosc 2001;15(8):898.
72. Honda G, Kurata M, Matsumura H, et al. Laparoscopy-assisted transduodenal papillectomy. Dig Surg 2010;27:123–6.
73. Hadjittofi C, Parisinos CA, Somri M, et al. Totally laparoscopic resection of a rare duodenal tumour. BMJ Case Rep 2012;2012 [pii:bcr0220125860].
74. Orsenigo E, Di Palo S, Vignali A, et al. Laparoscopic excision of duodenal schwannoma. Surg Endosc 2007;21(8):1454–6.
75. Poves I, Burdio F, Alonso S, et al. Laparoscopic pancreas-sparing subtotal duodenectomy. JOP 2011;12(5):62–5.
76. Dasari BVM, McKay D, Gardiner K. Laparoscopic versus Open surgery for small bowel Crohn's disease. Cochrane Database Syst Rev 2011;(1):CD006956.
77. Cirocchi R, Abraha I, Farinella E, et al. Laparoscopic versus open surgery in small bowel obstruction. Cochrane Database Syst Rev 2010;(2):CD007511.
78. Wexner SD, Johansen OB. Laparoscopic bowel resection: advantages and limitations. Ann Med 1992;24(2):105–10.

Minimally Invasive Colon Cancer Surgery

Katerina O. Wells, MD, MPH[a],*, Anthony Senagore, MD, MBA[b]

KEYWORDS

- Colon cancer • Surgical management • Minimally invasive • Laparoscopy
- Robotics • Colectomy • Outcomes

KEY POINTS

- The principles of oncologic resection include adequate lymph node harvest, proximal ligation of primary vasculature, and obtaining adequate distal and proximal margins.
- The addition of a total mesocolic excision may provide incremental improvements in outcomes.
- Preoperative planning must include tumor localization with distal margin tattooing, total colonic clearance, and operative risk assessment to determine the extent and appropriateness of the resection.
- Several randomized, controlled trials support the effectiveness of minimally invasive colectomy with improved short-term outcomes and noninferior oncologic outcomes compared with open surgery.

INTRODUCTION

Colon cancer is the second leading cause of cancer death in the United States.[1] With such a substantial impact on the population, innovation that advances the understanding of the pathogenesis and surgical and medical management of this disease continue to emerge. Surgical resection remains the most definitive tool in the treatment of colon cancer and the optimization of this modality through the use of minimally invasive techniques is quickly becoming the standard of care. Therefore, it is critical for the surgeon to have a clear understanding of the principles of oncologic resection in the minimally invasive setting. This article focuses on the surgical principles of resecting colon cancer. We review perioperative considerations, the technical aspects of a minimally invasive oncologic resection such as the importance of adequate lymph node harvest of more than 12 lymph nodes, ligation at the origin of primary vasculature

Disclosure: The authors have nothing to disclose.
[a] Department of Surgery, Baylor University Medical Center, 3409 Worth Street, Suite 640, Dallas, TX 75246, USA; [b] Department of Surgery, Western Michigan University, Homer Stryker School of Medicine, 1903 Western Michigan Avenue, Kalamazoo, MI 49008, USA
* Corresponding author.
E-mail address: Katerina.wells@bswhealth.org

surgonc.theclinics.com

(high ligation), obtaining adequate distal and proximal margins of 5 cm, and total mesocolic excision. We review the more recent concept of total mesocolic excision. We also review the current literature regarding oncologic and short-term outcomes of minimally invasive colon cancer surgery.

PREOPERATIVE PLANNING: TUMOR LOCALIZATION

Tumor localization before planned segmental resection is necessary, especially with a minimally invasive approach, when a tactile assessment is not an option for the palpation of a mass.[2] Errors in localization account for a 6.3% rate of alteration in preoperatively planned resection.[3] Endoscopic localization is highly inaccurate, with a 21% rate of error. This is especially the case for left-sided lesions and in patients with previous colonic resection, where anatomic landmarks are less recognizable.[4] India ink tattooing aids in intraoperative localization with a low risk of associated morbidity.[5] Although different techniques are used for tattooing, it is important to be consistent in the pattern of marking and to clearly document the method in the colonoscopy report. The authors recommend that tattoo be placed in 3 separate areas around the circumference of the lumen distal to the lesion. Submucosal infiltration is critical for identification because tattooing into the mesentery or transmurally into the peritoneal cavity can obscure accurate marking. Intraoperative colonoscopy with laparoscopic assistance can be used when preoperative localization measures fail.

PREOPERATIVE PLANNING: COLONIC CLEARANCE

Evaluation of the entire colon is also necessary to exclude synchronous lesions that can be present in 1% to 7% of patients with a primary colorectal cancer.[6]

Colonoscopy is accurate in the detection of primary and synchronous lesions with an estimated sensitivity and specificity of detecting malignancy of 85% and 95% and is the gold standard for colon clearance.[7] In the case of obstructing tumors that cannot be assessed endoscopically, computed tomography colonography is an accurate and well-tolerated method of noninvasive assessment that has replaced the barium enema. The sensitivity of computed tomography colonography in detecting proximal synchronous cancers is 100% with a specificity of 87.5% for cancers greater than 15 mm and a negative predictive value of close to 100%.[8] The localization error is low at 12% and computed tomography colonography is also 86% accurate for T staging, 70% accurate for N staging, and 94% accurate for the detection of intraabdominal metastatic disease.[9]

PREOPERATIVE PLANNING: PHYSIOLOGIC ASSESSMENT AND RISK STRATIFICATION AND ENHANCED RECOVERY AFTER SURGERY

A variety of risk stratification tools exist to determine a patient's risk of perioperative morbidity and mortality. The American Society of Anesthesia risk classification is the most pervasively used system for assessing risk; however, it is a broad assessment based on subjective criteria.[10] The American College of Surgeons National Surgical Quality Improvement Program risk calculator is a stratification tool developed and validated through aggregate multiinstitutional data from the National Surgical Quality Improvement Program. Risk assessments are most accurate at the surgeon-specific and institutional level and for average risk patients undergoing laparoscopic colectomy. Shortcomings of the American College of Surgeons National Surgical Quality Improvement Program calculator are related to the estimation of serious complication and estimation of risk in the comorbid patient.[11,12]

The Enhanced Recovery after Surgery Programs for colectomy are quickly becoming the standard for perioperative care. Fearon and colleagues[13] first introduced the Enhanced Recovery after Surgery as a bundle of interventions that work in concert to decrease postoperative stress, decrease recovery time, and decrease postoperative morbidity. Interventions emphasize a minimally invasive approach, mechanical and oral antibiotic bowel preparation, low-dose carbohydrate/balanced electrolyte preoperative drinks, the use of a transversus abdominus plane block, multimodality analgesia for reduction of narcotics use, and early mobilization and feeding. Enhanced Recovery after Surgery is a safe method of perioperative management that offers the advantage of fewer minor postoperative complications, decreased length of stay by a mean of 2.9 days without an increased risk of readmission as demonstrated in a 2011 Cochrane review.[14] Decreases in the length of stay and standardization of resource use also offer economic benefits.

PROCEDURAL APPROACH: ONCOLOGIC PRINCIPLES OF SURGICAL TECHNIQUE

Whatever the approach, minimally invasive or open, the basic principles as outlined by the National Comprehensive Cancer Network for oncologic resection of colon cancer include en bloc lymphadenectomy, ligation at the origin of feeding vessels (high ligation), and adequate proximal and distal resection margins. The purpose of proximal ligation of the primary feeding vessel is to maximize lymph node harvest and excise all potential mesenteric nodal disease owing to lateral migration of tumor cells within lymphatic drainage. High ligation is not associated with increased morbidity, with the benefit of increased disease-free survival with this technique.[15–18] A minimum of 12 nodes is necessary to be considered adequate lymphadenectomy for the purpose of accurate staging and improved overall and disease-specific survival.[19] Additionally, suspicious lymph nodes beyond the field of standard resection should be removed if possible, or at a minimum biopsied.[20]

A minimum of 5 cm is recommended for adequate proximal and distal margins. Resection length is also an indicator of adequate lymphadenectomy such that the a margin of less than 5 cm is associated with a significantly lower percentage of node-negative resections versus margins measuring greater than 5 cm (37% vs 51%) in a retrospective review by Rørvig and colleagues.[21] This finding suggests that shorter specimens may result in understaging owing to inadequate lymphadenectomy.

The technique of complete mesocolic excision is a newer concept advocating for the sharp dissection of the visceral fascia from the parietal fascia of the retroperitoneum and central ligation of the primary vasculature. This technique was first described by Hohenberger and colleagues,[22] who demonstrated a decrease in 5-year local recurrence and improvement in 5-year survival from 6.5% to 3.6% and 82.1% to 89.1%, respectively. The adoption of complete mesocolic excision is based on the learning from rectal cancer and the concept that cancers grow circumferentially and extend radially rather than longitudinally toward the embryologic planes of the specimen; therefore, the preservation of these planes of resection may decrease the risk of shedding tumor during dissection. Complete mesocolic excision with high ligation reports higher rates of lymph node harvest, and increased resection of extranodal tumor deposits and upstaging, which improve locoregional control and survival without reported added morbidity.[23] This technique has no confirmed benefit in prospective, randomized trials[24] and is not consistently adopted primarily because it is more technically demanding, requiring extensive dissection, especially so for right colectomy, in which the head of the pancreas and the anterior surface of the superior mesenteric vein and superior mesenteric artery are exposed to perform a true central ligation of the ileocolic and middle colic vasculature.[25]

PROCEDURAL APPROACH: RIGHT COLECTOMY

Right colectomy is the procedure recommended for tumors proximal to the proximal transverse colon. Principles of right-sided resection include abdominal exploration for distant disease, mobilization and medialization of the right colon and hepatic flexure to allow for resection and anastomosis, and high ligation of the ileocolic pedicle and right branch of the middle colic artery to ensure adequate lymph node retrieval. Using a laparoscopic approach, the peritoneal cavity is accessed with an open or closed technique. Once the abdomen is accessed and insufflated, all 4 quadrants should be explored to exclude obvious solid visceral involvement or peritoneal disease. There are several approaches to mobilizing the colon and its mesentery. The medial to lateral approach is commonly used in laparoscopic dissection. This approach accesses the retroperitoneum through the right colon mesentery on the caudad side of the ileocolic vessels (**Fig. 1**).

Once accessed, the duodenum is readily identified and dissection in the mesocolic plane allows the covering fascial layer over the retroperitoneum to be left intact over the duodenum (**Fig. 2**). This method then allows for the mobilization of the right colon off of the retroperitoneum in a medial to lateral direction. An inferior or posterior approach can be used in which the small bowel is eviscerated and reflected toward the right upper quadrant to expose the posterior aspect of the small bowel mesentery from the ligament of Treitz to the cecum. The retroperitoneum is accessed at the base of the ileal mesentery and the retromesocolic plane is developed, similar to the medial to lateral approach (**Fig. 3**). The disadvantage of this approach is the need for greater assistance in managing the large amount of bowel being mobilized.

In the case of a bulky or locally invasive tumor, the superior approach through the avascular attachments of the greater omentum to the transverse colon, allowing for initial mobilization of the proximal transverse colon so that the tumor can be addressed with 360° of freedom. The lateral to medial approach typically used in the open technique can also be used laparoscopically.

After mobilization and high ligation of the vascular pedicles, a 5-cm margin of the terminal ileum is obtained. The omentum overlying the segment of colon involved with tumor should also be excised with the specimen.

Typically, an extracorporeal resection and anastomosis is performed. However, with the availability of laparoscopic stapling devices and articulating graspers offered through robotic-assisted techniques, an intracorporal anastomosis is also feasible. Less mobilization is required of the transverse colon and a foreshortened middle colic

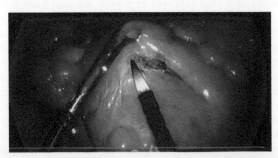

Fig. 1. Right colectomy. Accessing the retroperitoneum through the right colon mesentery.

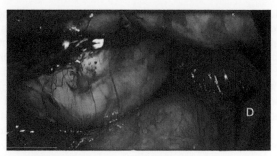

Fig. 2. Right colectomy. Development of the retromesocolic plane and reflection of the duodenum in to the retroperitoneum. D, duodenum.

pedicle. An ileocolic anastomosis can be accomplished via handsewn or stapled techniques with a side-to-side orientation to account for the luminal size mismatch.

PROCEDURAL APPROACH: TRANSVERSE COLON CANCERS

Cancers of the transverse colon are anatomically variable by the relationship of the tumor to 2 collateralizing vascular supplies with attendant variable lymphatic basins. Mobilization of the transverse colon is more technically challenging owing to the often foreshortened mesocolon overlying the pancreas and fragile middle colic vessels that are at risk for avulsion. For these reasons, extended right colectomy is recommended over left colectomy, such that the largely mobile terminal ileum can be positioned to the distal resection margin with relative ease. The procedure of right colectomy can be extended such that the greater omentum is divided to the distal transverse colon and the lesser sac exposed. After high ligation of the ileocolic vessels, the middle colic vessels are identified immediately adjacent to the ileocolic stump and high ligation of the middle colic vessels is performed. Care must be taken to ensure that the vessel to be divided clearly follows the course of the transverse colon mesentery to avoid inadvertent injury to the superior mesenteric artery. For distal transverse colon lesions, the left colic artery can be similarly ligated. The ileum is then mobilized for creation of the ileocolic anastomosis.

PROCEDURAL APPROACH: LEFT COLECTOMY

The basic steps of left colectomy for colon cancer include exploration of the abdomen to asses for distant disease, high ligation of inferior mesenteric artery (IMA) and the inferior mesenteric vein at the inferior border of the pancreas with visualization and

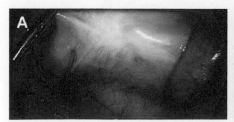
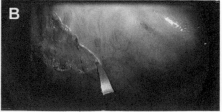

Fig. 3. (*A*) Right colectomy. Identifying the base of the ileal mesentery. (*B*) Right colectomy. Incising the peritoneum at the base of the ileal mesentery.

protection of the left ureter during these maneuvers, and complete mobilization of the left colon and splenic flexure to allow for a tension-free anastomosis.

Minimally invasive left colectomy can be performed through a straight or hand-assisted approach without any reported difference in short-term or oncologic outcomes. A Gelport is used for the hand port with placement based on operator preference. Common incisions for the handport include a suprapubic Pfannensteil, midline suprapubic, midline periumbilical, or left lower quadrant. Placing a handport in the suprapubic location allows for direct access to the pelvis for anastomotic creation and assessment. The hand port also serves as the extraction site for the specimen and the Gelport wound protector limits contamination and repetitive trauma to the abdominal wall.

The patient is placed in a dorsal lithotomy position to allow for operator standing room in between the legs and access to the perineum for transanal anastomosis and assessment. A medial to lateral approach begins with identification and manual retraction of the superior rectal artery off of the sacral promontory (**Fig. 4**).

The overlying peritoneum is incised from the sacral promontory to the IMA origin and the retromesocolic plane is propagated through blunt dissection. The left ureter is identified, preserving the overlying Toldts fascial layer in this process and swept downward into the retroperitoneum (**Fig. 5**).

If the ureter is not readily identifiable in this mesenteric window, the peritoneum can be incised in between the IMA and inferior mesenteric vein and the retroperitoneum similarly reflected to expose the ureter. If the ureter cannot be identified medially, the colon can be mobilized off of the retroperitoneum in a lateral to medial approach. Failure to identify the ureter after these maneuvers should prompt the placement of a ureteral stent or conversion to an open technique. After identification of the ureter, the IMA can be safely ligated at its origin using a laparoscopic energy device (**Fig. 6**). This step allows for the further development of the retromesocolic plane cephalad to the inferior border of the pancreas and laterally to the white line of Toldt. The inferior mesenteric vein can then be divided at the inferior border of the pancreas (**Fig. 7**). The remaining white line of Toldt and splenocolic attachments can be divided to complete the mobilization of the flexure.

Various approaches can be used for proximal and distal transection. This procedure can be performed in an open approach through the handport. Alternatively, the distal rectum can be divided laparoscopically and the proximal colon transected upon extraction of the specimen. Alternatively, resection and anastomosis can be performed intracorporeally. The proximal point of transection should be one that that is well-perfused, reaches the pelvis without tension, and satisfies a 5-cm margin from

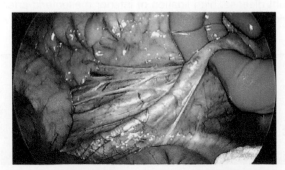

Fig. 4. Left colectomy. Manual retraction of the superior rectal artery off of the sacral promontory.

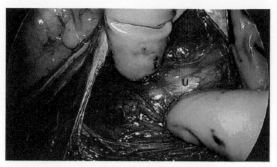

Fig. 5. Left colectomy. Identification of the ureter. U, ureter.

the tumor mass. The point of distal transection should also be at least 5 cm from the tumor mass or further to allow for transection at the top of the rectum to avoid anastomosis to the less compliant sigmoid colon.

The double staple technique in either an end-to-end or side-to-end coloproctostomy is most easily performed. A stapled side-to-side functional end-to-end technique can also be used provided enough length is available or if an ileo-rectal anastomosis is performed. The end-to-end anastomosis anvil is inserted to the proximal bowel and secured in a purse-string fashion. It is important to ensure that no gaps occur in the purse-string and that the mucosal edges are well-everted against the anvil. The end-to-end anastomosis stapler is then inserted transanally to the level of distal transection. In the case of resistance with passage of the stapler, the rectum should be evaluated for stricture, adhesion, or valves that may limit passage to the staple line. If this situation is encountered, lysis of adhesion with rectal mobilization is needed to straighten the rectum to allow passage of the end-to-end anastomosis to top of the rectal stump. The spike of the end-to-end anastomosis is deployed through the top of the distal point of transection and mated to the anvil. Caution should be taken to ensure that the proximal bowel is not under torsion or tension and that no intervening tissue is entrapped in the staple line before firing.

PROCEDURAL APPROACH: ANASTOMOTIC TESTING

Anastomotic testing is recommended after the creation of the left-sided anastomosis, and doing so is associated with a decreased incidence of leak. Routine intraoperative sigmoidoscopy or rigid proctoscopy can be performed to directly visualize the

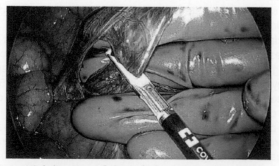

Fig. 6. Left colectomy. High ligation of the inferior mesenteric artery.

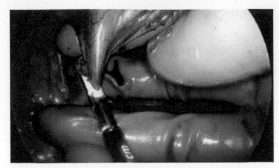

Fig. 7. Left colectomy. Division of the inferior mesenteric vein at the inferior border of the pancreas.

anastomosis and assess for integrity and bleeding. The rate of positive air leak after anastomotic testing is relatively high, emphasizing the need for assessment and intervention in the case of positive leak. Kamal and colleagues[26] prospectively reviewed 415 patients, in which 15 of 17 patients found to have an endoscopic abnormality had a positive air leak test. The rate of clinically evident leak after revision in these patients resulted in an overall leak rate of 2.1%. In a retrospective review of 998 patients undergoing colorectal anastomosis, the overall leak rate was 4.8%, whereas the rate of clinically evident leaks was significantly lower at 3.8% versus 7.7% after negative air leak testing. In comparing the method of repair for positive air leaks, anastomotic revision or proximal diversion were more effective at preventing clinically evident leaks compared with suture repair alone.[27]

CLINICAL RESULTS IN THE LITERATURE: ONCOLOGIC OUTCOMES

Over the last 3 decades, several randomized, controlled trials have supported the effectiveness of minimally invasive colectomy for colon cancer with improved short-term outcomes and noninferior oncologic outcomes compared with open surgery. The COST trial is a multicenter trial of 48 centers designed with the primary objective of demonstrating noninferiority in the primary outcomes of time to recurrence and secondary outcomes of disease-free and overall survival between laparoscopic-assisted versus open colectomy using a noninferiority design. Overall recurrence, 5-year disease-free survival, and 5-year overall survival were similar between groups. To address the concern of port site seeding in laparoscopic colectomy, the rate of wound recurrence was similar between groups and exceedingly low (open: wound 0.5% vs laparoscopic: wound 0.9%).[28,29] The COST trial also demonstrated faster perioperative recovery, shorter length of stay, and lower use of parenteral and oral analgesics after laparoscopic surgery.[30]

The COLOR trial is a multicenter trial involving 29 centers across Europe with the primary outcomes of 3-year disease-free survival. Pathologic oncologic criteria were similar between groups. The hazard ratio for disease survival of open versus laparoscopic colectomy was 0.92 (95% confidence interval [CI], 0.74–1.15) with an overall survival difference of 2.4% (95% CI, -2.1 to 7.0) that was considered clinically acceptable based on a prespecified noninferiority boundary of 7%.[31,32]

The outcomes of the UK MRC CLASICC similarly compared laparoscopic with open colectomy and proctectomy across 27 centers in the UK and found no statistically significant differences in pathologic criteria, overall survival, disease-free survival, and recurrence. However, conversion was associated with decreased overall and disease-free survival regardless of surgeon experience (overall survival: hazard ratio, 2.28 [95% CI, 1.47–3.53]; disease-free survival: hazard ratio, 2.20 [95 CI, 1.31–3.67]), suggesting that tumor biology attributed to this increase and advanced tumors may be less suited to a minimally invasive approach.[33–35]

CLINICAL RESULTS IN THE LITERATURE: SHORT-TERM OUTCOMES

Laparoscopy also offers clear short-term benefits compared with open surgery. In a 2005 Cochrane review of 25 randomized, controlled trials including the landmark studies outlined elsewhere in this article, laparoscopic colectomy offered advantages in lower postoperative pain scores (weighted mean difference, −12.9; 95% CI, −19.8 to -6.0; $P = .0002$), shorter length of postoperative ileus by 0.9 to 1.0 day (weighted mean difference, 1.03; 95% CI, −1.30 to −0.76; $P<.0001$), and fewer postoperative complications (18.2% laparoscopic vs 23.0% open) with an overall relative risk of 0.72 (95% CI, 0.55–0.95; $P = .02$).[36] In a retrospective review of the National Cancer Database, laparoscopy also afforded improved 30-day mortality (1.3% vs 2.3%; $P<.001$), shorter length of stay (median 5 vs 6 days; incident rate ratio, 0.83; 95% CI, 0.8–0.84; $P<.001$), and higher rates of adjuvant chemotherapy use in stage III patients (72.3% vs 67.0%; $P<.001$).[37] This last outcome measure may be a more valuable measure of short-term benefit because of its potential to translate into long-term oncologic advantage.

CLINICAL RESULTS IN THE LITERATURE: ROBOTIC-ASSISTED COLECTOMY

Robotic surgery has seen greater use in colorectal surgery owing to the perceived benefits of articulating instruments and multi-instrument retraction and maneuverability over in-line laparoscopic instruments for laparoscopic proctectomy. The comfort of the robotic console over bedside operative also results in less surgeon fatigue compared with laparoscopy.[38] Noninferiority of this technique for rectal cancer surgery has been supported in several randomized, controlled trials, with the caveat of longer operative time and significant increases in operating room costs.[39–42] As newer models allow for multiquadrant dissection, its application for colon cancer is considered. In systematic review of the available literature, robotic colectomy for cancer is comparably safe and feasible as laparoscopic colectomy, with similar rates of postoperative length of stay, morbidity, and mortality.[43] In metaanalysis of 14 studies comparing laparoscopic with robotic colectomy, the operating time for robotic colectomy significantly exceeded laparoscopic colectomy by a mean difference of 49 minutes (95% CI, 36.78–61.72; $P<.00001$) translating to significantly greater overall costs in comparison with standard techniques.[44] In the absence of randomized, controlled trials, the role of current robotic technology for colectomy remains unclear.

SUMMARY

Colon cancer is one of the most common cancers in the United States and advances in colon cancer surgery continue to emerge. Regardless of innovation, colectomy for cancer adheres to the oncologic principles of adequate lymphadenectomy, high ligation of primary vessels, adequate longitudinal margins, and possibly the addition of a complete mesocolic excision. For left-sided anastomoses, anastomotic testing is necessary to decrease the rate of clinically apparent leak. Minimally invasive colectomy for colon cancer is established as a feasible and safe technique for the surgical management of colon cancer as supported by multiple randomized, controlled trials. Moreover, laparoscopy affords greater short-term benefits of less pain and shorter length of stay compared with open surgery. The role of robotics in colon cancer surgery is supported; however, further clarity is needed regarding the cost-benefit of this technique.

REFERENCES

1. National Cancer Institute, surveillance, epidemiology, and end results program. Cancer stat facts: colorectal cancer. Available at: http://seer.cancer.gov/statfacts/html/colorect.html. Accessed February 1, 2018.

2. Cho YB, Lee WY, Yun HR, et al. Tumor localization for laparoscopic colorectal surgery. World J Surg 2007;31:1491–5.

3. Johnstone M, Moug S. The accuracy of colonoscopic localisation of colorectal tumours: a prospective, multi-centered observational study. Scott Med J 2014; 59(2):85–90.

4. Piscatelli N, Hyman N, Osler T. Localizing colorectal cancer by colonoscopy. Arch Surg 2005;140(10):932–5.

5. Botoman VA, Pietro M, Thirlby RC. Localization of colonic lesions with endoscopic tattoo. Dis Colon Rectum 1994;37:775–6.

6. Mulder SA, Kranse R, Damhuis RA, et al. Prevalence and prognosis of synchronous colorectal cancer: a Dutch population-based study. Cancer Epidemiol 2011;35:442–7.

7. Nishihara R, Wu K, Lochhead P, et al. Long-term colorectal-cancer incidence and mortality after lower endoscopy. N Engl J Med 2013;369(12):1095–105.

8. Park SH, Lee JH, Lee SS, et al. CT colonography for detection and characterisation of synchronous proximal colonic lesions in patients with stenosing colorectal cancer. Gut 2012;61(12):1716–22.

9. Kim JH, Kim WH, Kim TI, et al. Incomplete colonoscopy in patients with occlusive colorectal cancer: usefulness of CT colonography according to tumor location. Yonsei Med J 2007;48:934.

10. Wolters U, Wolf T, Stützer H, et al. ASA classification and perioperative variables as predictors of postoperative outcome. Br J Anaesth 1996;77(2):217–22.

11. Cologne KG, Keller DS, Liwanag L, et al. Use of the American College of Surgeons NSQIP surgical risk calculator for laparoscopic colectomy: how good is it and how can we improve it? J Am Coll Surg 2015;220(3):281–6.

12. Cohen ME, Bilimoria KY, Yo CY, et al. Development of an American College of Surgeons national surgery quality improvement program: morbidity and mortality risk calculator for colorectal surgery. J Am Coll Surg 2009;208(6):1009–16.

13. Fearon KC, Ljungqvist O, Von Meyenfeldt M, et al. Enhanced recovery after surgery: a consensus review of clinical care for patients undergoing colonic resection. Clin Nutr 2005;24(3):466–77.

14. Spanjersberg WR, Reurings J, Keus F, et al. Fast track surgery versus conventional recovery strategies for colorectal surgery. Cochrane Database Syst Rev 2011;(2):CD007635.

15. Read TE, Mutch MG, Chang BW, et al. Locoregional recurrence and survival after curative resection of adenocarcinoma of the colon. J Am Coll Surg 2002;195(1): 33–40.

16. Chin CC, Yeh CY, Tang R, et al. The oncologic benefit of high ligation of the inferior mesenteric artery in the surgical treatment of rectal or sigmoid colon cancer. Int J Colorectal Dis 2008;23(8):783–8.

17. Kanemitsu Y, Hirai T, Komori K, et al. Survival benefit of high ligation of the inferior mesenteric artery in sigmoid colon or rectal cancer surgery. Br J Surg 2006;93(5): 609–15.

18. Matsuda K, Hotta T, Takifuji K, et al. Randomized clinical trial of defaecatory function after anterior resection for rectal cancer with high versus low ligation of the inferior mesenteric artery. Br J Surg 2015;102(5):501–8.

19. Voyer TE, Sigurdson ER, Hanlon AL, et al. Colon cancer survival is associated with increasing number of lymph nodes analyzed: a secondary survey of intergroup trial INT-0089. J Clin Oncol 2003;21(15):2912–9.

20. Benson AB, Venook AP, Bekai-Saab T, et al. Colon cancer, version 3.2014. J Natl Compr Canc Netw 2014;12(7):1028–59.

21. Rørvig S, Schlesinger N, Mårtensson NL, et al. Is the longitudinal margin of carcinoma-bearing colon resections a neglected parameter? Clin Colorectal Cancer 2014;13(1):68–72.

22. Hohenberger W, Weber K, Matzel K, et al. Standardized surgery for colonic cancer: complete mesocolic excision and central ligation-technical notes and outcome. Colorectal Dis 2009;11(4):354–64.

23. Galizia G, Lieto E, De Vita F, et al. Is complete mesocolic excision with central vascular ligation safe and effective in the surgical treatment of right-sided colon cancers? A prospective study. Int J Colorectal Dis 2014;29(1):89–97.

24. Emmanuel A, Haji A. Complete mesocolic excision and extended (D3) lymphadenectomy for colonic cancer: is it worth that extra effort? A review of the literature. Int J Colorectal Dis 2016;31(4):797–804.

25. Bae SU, Saklani AP, Lim DR, et al. Laparoscopic-assisted versus open complete mesocolic excision and central vascular ligation for right-sided colon cancer. Ann Surg Oncol 2014;21(7):2288–94.

26. Kamal T, Pai A, Velchuru V, et al. Should anastomotic assessment with flexible sigmoidoscopy be routine following laparoscopic restorative left colorectal resection? Colorectal Dis 2015;17(2):160–4.

27. Ricciardi R, Roberts PL, Marcello PW, et al. Anastomotic leak testing after colorectal resection: what are the data? Arch Surg 2009;144(5):407–11.

28. Clinical Outcomes of Surgical Therapy Study Group, Nelson H, Sargent DJ, Wieand HS, et al. A comparison of laparoscopically assisted and open colectomy for colon cancer. N Engl J Med 2004;350(20):2050–9.

29. Fleshman J, Sargent DJ, Green E, et al. Laparoscopic colectomy for cancer is not inferior to open surgery based on 5-year data from the COST study group trial. Ann Surg 2007;246(4):655–62.

30. Stucky CC, Pockaj BA, Novotny PJ, et al. Long-term follow-up and individual item analysis of quality of life assessments related to laparoscopic-assisted colectomy in the COST trial 93-46-53 (INT 0146). Ann Surg Oncol 2011;18(9):2422–31.

31. Veldkamp R, Kuhry E, Hop WC, et al. Laparoscopic surgery versus open surgery for colon cancer: short-term outcomes of a randomised trial. Lancet Oncol 2005; 6(7):477–84.

32. The Colon Cancer Laparoscopic or Open Resection Study Group. Survival after laparoscopic surgery versus open surgery for colon cancer: long-term outcome of a randomised clinical trial. Lancet Oncol 2009;10(1):44–52.

33. Kuhry E, Bonjer HJ, Haglind E, et al. Impact of hospital case volume on short-term outcome after laparoscopic operation for colonic cancer. Surg Endosc 2005;19:687–92.

34. Guillou PJ, Quirke P, Thorpe H, et al. Short-term endpoints of conventional versus laparoscopic-assisted surgery in patients with colorectal cancer (MRC CLASICC trial). Lancet 2005;365(9472):1718–26.
35. Jayne DG, Thorpe HC, Copeland J, et al. Five-year follow-up of the Medical Research Council CLASICC trial of laparoscopically assisted versus open surgery for colorectal cancer. Br J Surg 2010;97(11):1638–45.
36. Schwenk W, Haase O, Neudecker J, et al. Short term benefits for laparoscopic colorectal resection. Cochrane Database Syst Rev 2005;(3):CD003145.
37. Zheng Z, Jemal A, Lin CC, et al. Comparative effectiveness of laparoscopy vs open colectomy among nonmetastatic colon cancer patients: an analysis using the national cancer data base. J Natl Cancer Inst 2015;107(3) [pii:dju491].
38. Pigazzi A, Ellenhorn JD, Ballantyne GH, et al. Robotic-assisted laparoscopic low anterior resection with total mesorectal excision for rectal cancer. Surg Endosc 2006;20(10):1521–5.
39. Kim MJ, Park SC, Park JW, et al. Robot-assisted versus laparoscopic surgery for rectal cancer: a phase ii open label prospective randomized controlled trial. Ann Surg 2017. https://doi.org/10.1097/SLA.0000000000002321.
40. Saklani AP, Lim DR, Hur H, et al. Robotic versus laparoscopic surgery for mid–low rectal cancer after neoadjuvant chemoradiation therapy: comparison of oncologic outcomes. Int J Colorectal Dis 2013;28(12):1689–98.
41. Baek SJ, Al-Asari S, Jeong DH, et al. Robotic versus laparoscopic coloanal anastomosis with or without intersphincteric resection for rectal cancer. Surg Endosc 2013;27(11):4157–63.
42. Collinson FJ, Jayne DG, Pigazzi A, et al. An international, multicentre, prospective, randomised, controlled, unblinded, parallel-group trial of robotic-assisted versus standard laparoscopic surgery for the curative treatment of rectal cancer. Int J Colorectal Dis 2011;27(2):233–41.
43. Fung AKY, Aly EH. Robotic colonic surgery: is it advisable to commence a new learning curve? Dis Colon Rectum 2013;56(6):786–96.
44. Chang YS, Wang JX, Chang DW. ScienceDirect. J Surg Res 2015;195(2):465–74.

Minimally Invasive Surgery for Locally Advanced Rectal Cancer

Katerina O. Wells, MD, MPH, Walter R. Peters, MD, MBA*

KEYWORDS

- Proctectomy • Total mesorectal excision • Laparoscopy • Robotic surgery
- Transanal TME • Minimally invasive surgery • Rectal cancer

KEY POINTS

- The quality of surgical resection, defined as performance of a total mesorectal excision with negative circumferential margins, is an important determinant of prognosis.
- Minimally invasive surgery offers patients with colorectal cancer short-term benefits, including decreased pain, shorter postoperative hospital stays, and shorter time to initiation of adjuvant chemotherapy.
- Minimally invasive resection of rectal cancer is technically difficult, especially for cancers in the low rectum. Identification of the optimal technique and instrumentation is in evolution.
- Randomized controlled trials of laparoscopic versus open surgery for rectal cancer have yielded different conclusions regarding oncologic equivalence due to differences in study design and patient characteristics.
- Surgeons should treat rectal cancer within the model of a multidisciplinary team with the capability to audit the quality and outcomes of the care provided.

INTRODUCTION

Minimally invasive surgery revolutionized the field of colorectal surgery, beginning with the first reported laparoscopic segmental colectomies in 1990. Patients and surgeons were initially drawn to the potential short-term benefits, including decreased pain, improved cosmesis, shorter hospital stay, and a quicker recovery; however, it was quickly noted that there was a significant learning curve for these complex, multiquadrant procedures. Enthusiasm was further dampened by early reports of tumor recurrence following laparoscopic colon cancer surgery, leading to questions about

Disclosure: The authors have nothing to disclose.
Division of Colon and Rectal Surgery, Baylor University Medical Center, 3500 Gaston Avenue, Dallas, TX 75246, USA
* Corresponding author.
E-mail address: Walter.Peters@BSWHealth.org

the appropriateness of minimally invasive surgery for the curative resection of colorectal cancer. These concerns were partially put to rest with the publication of the COST Trial in 2004, which found that laparoscopic colectomy was noninferior when compared with open surgery for the treatment of colon cancer.[1] This study excluded patients with cancer of the rectum, however, leaving surgeons to question whether the results could be extrapolated to the treatment of locally advanced rectal cancer.

The surgical treatment of rectal cancer differs from the treatment of colon cancer in several important ways. Surgery is more often performed in the setting of multimodal therapy, with surgery, chemotherapy, and radiation therapy used in a variety of treatment algorithms. The recommended treatment, including surgical approach, varies based on clinical staging. The surgical procedures are generally more difficult, due to the confines of the pelvis, the limitations of exposure in the deep pelvis and the risk of injury to adjacent structures. These differences between the treatment of colon cancer and rectal cancer necessitated further study before embracing minimally invasive surgery for rectal cancer.

TOTAL MESORECTAL EXCISION

The emphasis on surgical technique as a determinant of local recurrence and survival can be attributed to the work of Heald and colleagues[2] and Quirk and colleagues.[3] Heald and colleagues[2] hypothesized that local recurrence often resulted from microscopic tumor deposits within the mesorectum distal to the primary tumor. They proposed that excision of the entire mesorectum, total mesorectal excision (TME), would reduce the rate of local recurrence.[2] Quirk and colleagues[3] demonstrated that traditional pathologic evaluation of rectal cancer specimens ignored the importance of the circumferential radial margin (CRM).[3] They developed and promoted pathologic emphasis on evaluation of the completeness of the mesorectal excision and the status of the radial margins.

The importance of this emphasis on the adequacy of resection was underscored by studies from Europe that demonstrated improved rates of local recurrence following formal efforts to train surgeons in the technique of TME.[4] In 1993, McFarlane and colleagues[5] reported a personal series of patients with stage II and III rectal cancer treated by TME alone. Local recurrence and survival compared favorably with a contemporaneous randomized controlled trial of surgery, followed by radiation or radiation plus chemotherapy.[5]

TME requires circumferential sharp dissection of the contents of the mesorectal fascia, beginning at the sacral promontory, and proceeding to the pelvic floor. The pelvic splanchnic nerves and ureters are positioned laterally and must be protected from injury. The anterolateral ligaments containing the middle hemorrhoidal vessels and splanchnic nerve branches are identified with medial traction of the rectum and should be divided away from the lateral pelvic sidewall to prevent damage to the nerve trunks. Sharp or cautery devices allow for precise dissection. For posterior tumors, anterior dissection begins immediately behind the Denonvilliers fascia, preserving nerves of sexual function traveling to the bladder, prostate, and sexual organs. For anterior tumors, dissection includes the Denonvilliers fascia, exposing the seminal vesicles or posterior vaginal wall to ensure a clear anterior margin at the expense of potential damage to the nerves of urogenital function. Further dissection is guided by the extent of the cancer as seen on preoperative imaging. Dissection may continue over the surface of the levators into the upper anal canal if ultralow resection is needed, or through the levators if an extralevator abdominoperineal resection is indicated. The completed TME is a circumferentially encased fascial envelope with a bilobed configuration of the posterior mesorectum. In tumor-specific TME (TSTME), the mesorectum is transected at the appropriate distal margin at a right angle to the axis of the mesorectum without coning of the mesorectum in the vicinity of the tumor. The integrity of the mesorectum is graded by the pathologist as complete, nearly complete, and incomplete. Complete and near-complete excisions yield similar clinical outcomes and are considered acceptable technical results. Incomplete mesorectal excisions carry the potential risk of retained mesorectal tissue with local nodal recurrence in the pelvis.

CLINICAL TRIALS OF LAPAROSCOPIC TOTAL MESORECTAL EXCISION

Since the late 1990s, nonrandomized studies have supported the use of laparoscopic surgery for rectal cancer.[6–8] There is also now a body of randomized controlled trials reported in the past decade evaluating the surgical and oncologic efficacy of this technique (**Table 1**). The UK MRC Conventional vs Laparoscopic-Assisted Surgery in Colorectal Cancer (CLASICC) Trial,[9,10] Comparison of OPEN vs Laparoscopic Surgery for mid or low Rectal Cancer after Neoadjuvant Chemoradiotherapy (COREAN) Trial,[11,12] Colorectal Cancer Laparoscopic or OPEN Resection (COLOR) II Trial,[13] Z6051Trial,[14] and Australian Laparoscopic Compared with open Low Anterior Resection Trial (ALaCaRTE)[15] are randomized rectal cancer trials comparing open to minimally invasive surgery and have reported seemingly conflicting results. This apparent conflict may be explained by significant differences in study design and patient characteristics.

Conventional vs Laparoscopic-Assisted Surgery in Colorectal Cancer Trial

The earliest randomized controlled, multicenter trial is the UK MRC CLASICC trial, which reported short-term outcomes in 2005. The trial enrolled patients with both colon and rectal cancer requiring both curative and palliative resections. Patients were randomized 2:1 to receive laparoscopic or open resection with no attempt to standardize surgical technique. In subset analysis of patients with rectal cancer (50% of the study population) circumferential radial margin (CRM) positivity was greater in patients undergoing a laparoscopic anterior resection (12%) than in the open group (6%), but this difference was not statistically significant. The conversion rate of 34% for patients with rectal cancer, and a steadily decreasing conversion rate throughout the trial, suggested that many surgeons were still in a relatively early portion of the learning curve. The short-term results led the investigators to conclude that the results did not justify the routine use of the laparoscopic approach for rectal cancer.[9] In a subsequent report, a trend toward improved early survival was observed in the laparoscopic group; however, 3-year overall survival (OS), disease-free survival (DFS), and local recurrence (9.7% laparoscopic vs 10.1% open) were similar. The investigators concluded that the data now supported the use of laparoscopic surgery for both colon and rectal cancer.[10]

Comparison of Open vs Laparoscopic Surgery for mid or low Rectal Cancer after Neoadjuvant Chemoradiotherapy Trial

The COREAN trial, published in 2014, was a noninferiority study of 340 patients conducted at 3 institutions in Korea. The trial included only patients with clinical stage II and III mid to low rectal cancers (0–9 cm from the anal verge) who had all received preoperative chemoradiation. They were randomized 1:1 to laparoscopic versus open resection. The primary endpoint was 3-year DFS, using a noninferiority margin of 15%. Conversion was exceedingly low at 1.2% with acceptable TME in 92% (laparoscopic) and 88% (open), $P = .41$. There was no difference in CRM positivity between laparoscopic (2.9%) or open (4.1%) techniques, $P = .77$.[11] Of note, the mean body

Table 1
Major RCTs of laparoscopic versus open TME

Study	Type	n	Stages	Preoperative XRT	Location		Endpoint	Conclusion
CLASICC,[9] 2005	RCT	794	Colon and rectum Stage I–IV	Not reported	Not reported		Multiple	"…impaired short-term outcomes after laparoscopic-assisted anterior resection for cancer of the rectum do not yet justify its routine use."
CLASICC,[10] 2012							OS, DFS, LR	"Long-term results continue to support the use of laparoscopic surgery for both colonic and rectal cancer."
COREAN,[12] 2014	RCT noninferiority 15% margin	340	Rectum (0–9 cm) Stage II–III	100%	0–3 cm 3–6 cm 6–9 cm	21% 39% 41%	3-y DFS	"…laparoscopic resection for locally advanced rectal cancer after preoperative chemoradiotherapy provides similar outcomes for disease-free survival as open resection, thus justifying its use."
COLOR II,[13] 2015	RCT noninferiority 5% margin	1044	Rectum (0–15 cm) Stage I–III	59%	0–5 cm 5–10 cm 10–15 cm	29% 39% 32%	3-y LR	"…laparoscopic surgery is as safe and effective as open surgery in patients with rectal cancers without invasion of adjacent tissues."
Z6051,[14] 2015	RCT noninferiority 6% margin	486	Rectum (0–12 cm) Stage II–III	100%	0–5 cm 5–10 cm 10–15 cm	51% 35% 14%	Composite (neg DM, neg CRM, complete or near-complete TME)	"…the findings do not support the use of laparoscopic resection in these patients."
ALaCaRT,[15] 2015	RCT noninferiority 8% margin	475	Rectum (0–15 cm) Stage I–IV	50%	0–5 cm 5–10 cm 10–15 cm	35% 43% 22%	Composite (neg DM, neg CRM, complete TME)	"…these findings do not provide sufficient evidence for the routine use of laparoscopic surgery."

Abbreviations: CRM, circumferential resection margin; DFS, disease-free survival; DM, distal margin; LR, local recurrence; neg, negative; OS, overall survival; RCT, randomized controlled trial; TME, total mesorectal excision; XRT, radiation therapy.

mass index (BMI) of 24 and the exceedingly low conversion rate suggest the results may not be generalizable to western populations. Stage-specific analysis showed similar DFS, OS, and local recurrence rates between groups.[12]

Colorectal Cancer Laparoscopic or Open Resection II Trial

The COLOR II trial (Colorectal Cancer Laparoscopic or Open Resection), reported in 2015, was a noninferiority trial conducted in 30 centers across Europe and including 1044 patients with clinical stage I to III rectal cancer, defined as within 15 cm of the anal verge. Patients were randomized in a 2:1 fashion to laparoscopic versus open resection. The conversion rate was 16%, reflecting increasing familiarity with the laparoscopic approach. Thirty-three percent of the laparoscopic cohort had pathologic stage I disease, 32% of tumors were in the upper rectum (10–15 cm), only 29% were in the low rectum (0–5) and just 59% of patients received preoperative radiotherapy. The primary endpoint of 3-year local recurrence was within the noninferiority margin of 5% and comparable between cohorts at 5%. Three-year OS and 3-year DFS were similar with improved DFS among stage II patients treated with laparoscopic resection. Pathologic evaluation found acceptable TME (complete or nearly complete mesorectum) in 92% of laparoscopic resections and 94% of open, 100% negative distal margins, and 10% positive CRM for both groups. However, CRM positivity for open resection of low rectal cancers was surprisingly high at 22%. The trial concluded that laparoscopic TME in laparoscopic surgery is as safe and effective as open surgery in patients with rectal cancers without invasion of adjacent tissues.[13]

A SURROGATE PATHOLOGIC ENDPOINT

The concept of using a surrogate oncologic endpoint was developed for 2 subsequent randomized trials of minimally invasive surgery for rectal cancer. To have adequate power to detect relatively small differences of outcomes, rectal cancer surgery trials require large numbers of patients. Even with multiple institutions participating, trials may take years to accrue adequate numbers of patients. An oncologic endpoint, such as 3-year survival, necessitates further delay as the patients are observed for this outcome. If, instead, the endpoint consisted of a composite of pathologic features known to correlate with oncologic outcomes, such as local recurrence or survival, the endpoint could be determined immediately, thus allowing earlier analysis of outcomes. For the US Z6051 trial and the Australian ALaCaRT trial, the composite endpoint of a satisfactory outcome was defined as a negative distal margin, a negative CRM, and a mesorectal resection specimen graded as complete or nearly complete.

Z6051

American College of Surgeons Oncology Group (ACOSOG) Z6051 was a randomized noninferiority trial conducted at 35 centers in the United States and Canada. As in the COST study, all participating surgeons were credentialed by review of operative reports and a video demonstrating the surgeon's technique. Patients with clinical stage II or III rectal cancer within 12 cm of the anal verge were eligible. After completing neoadjuvant therapy, patients were randomized to open (n = 222) or laparoscopic (n = 242) TME. More than half of the patients in the laparoscopic arm had cancer located in the low rectum (0–5 cm above the anal verge). The "laparoscopic" arm included patients who underwent a hand-assisted laparoscopic resection (17%) or robotic resection (14%). The conversion rate of 11.3% and the anastomotic leak rate of 2.2% validate the expertise of the credentialed surgeons. Successful resection as determined by the composite endpoint (negative distal margin, negative CRM, and complete or near-complete TME specimen) was 81.7% in the laparoscopic group and 86.9% in the open group, for a 5.3% difference. The rate of negative CRM was lower in the laparoscopic group (87.9% vs 92.3%), as was the rate of complete or nearly complete TME (92.1% vs 95.1%). Although the differences in individual components were not significant, the 95% confidence interval (CI) around the 5.3% difference did not support noninferiority (difference −5.3%; 1-sided 95% CI −10.8% to infinity; $P = .41$). The investigators concluded that this trial, using the composite pathologic endpoint, could not support the use of laparoscopic resection for patients with stage II/III rectal cancer until the clinical oncologic outcomes could be determined.[14]

Australian Laparoscopic Compared with Open Low Anterior Resection Trial

ALaCaRT was also reported in 2015. ALaCaRT was a randomized, noninferiority trial intended to model the protocol of ACOSOG Z6051 by using a similar composite pathologic endpoint as a surrogate for clinical oncologic outcomes. Unlike Z6051, which considered both complete and nearly complete TME as successful, ALaCaRT required a complete specimen as a marker of success. The trial was conducted by 26 accredited surgeons from 24 centers in Australia and New Zealand. ALaCaRT enrolled patients with clinical stage I to IV with tumors up to 15 cm from the anal verge. Fewer patients (35%) had low rectal cancers (<5 cm) and only 50% of patients underwent preoperative radiotherapy. The margin for noninferiority was 8%. The quality of surgery was high, with a conversion rate of only 9% and no significant difference in the short-term outcomes between groups. Successful resection as determined by the composite endpoint was 82% in the laparoscopic group and 89% in the open group with a difference in risk of −7.0%. As in the Z6051 trial, the laparoscopic cohort had lower rates of CRM negativity (93% vs 97%) and complete TME (87% vs 92%) than the open cohort. Although the difference of −7% was less than the established margin of −8%, the 95% CI was −12.4% to infinity ($P = .38$), which failed to establish noninferiority. Based on these findings, laparoscopic rectal resection cannot be considered noninferior to open surgery and caution is needed before uniformly applying this technique for the management of rectal cancer.[15] Long-term oncologic outcomes are currently being acquired.

RECONCILING THE DIFFERENCES

Both the Z6051 trial and ALaCaRT have yet to report long-term clinical oncologic outcomes. It may well be that the failure to establish noninferiority based on the composite surrogate endpoint will not translate into significantly different clinical outcomes. A meta-analysis of the outcomes of COLOR II, COREAN, ALaCaRT, and ACOSOG Z6051 is anticipated and may provide more clarity. Still, it is disconcerting that highly motivated, experienced, accredited surgeons in 2 major trials could not clearly demonstrate noninferiority of the laparoscopic technique. The lack of concordance between the reassuring findings of CLASICC and COLOR II, and the unsettling results of Z6051 and ALaCaRT, may be partly explained by the higher percentage of low rectal cancers in the latter two studies. Dissection becomes progressively more difficult in the lower pelvis and may expose the shortcomings of nonarticulating laparoscopic instruments. Another difference is the greater use of neoadjuvant therapy in the Z6051 study. ALaCaRT noted a −14% difference in success rate of resections in patients who had preoperative radiotherapy, although the difference did not achieve significance. It is likely that the 5 studies described previously have shown that laparoscopic surgery is safe and effective for upper rectal cancers, but differences in the treatment of low rectal cancers should raise caution.

SHORT-TERM OUTCOMES

The short-term benefits of laparoscopy are clearly demonstrated. In a 2014 Cochrane review of 14 studies and 3528 patients with rectal cancer, there is moderate-quality evidence that laparoscopy affords shorter hospital stay by 2 days (95% CI −3.22 to −1.10), shorter time to defecation by almost 1 day (95% CI −1.17 to −0.54). with fewer wound infections (odds ratio [OR] 0.68; 95% CI 0.50–0.93), bleeding complications (OR 0.30; 95% CI 0.10–0.93), and similar 30-day morbidity (OR 0.94; 95% CI 0.8–1.1) compared with open resection. Laparoscopic resection also afforded lower analgesic use, pain scores, and length of incision was significantly shorter by 12 cm (mean difference[MD] −12.83; 95% CI −14.87 to −10.80).[8] In a more recent meta-analysis by Zheng and colleagues,[16] including 38 studies and 13,408 patients, similar benefits of decreased complications and early recovery with laparoscopic technique were realized at the expense of significantly increased operative times (MD 37.23 minutes; 95% CI 28.88–45.57, P<.0001).

In addition to the immediate surgical advantages, Strouch and colleagues[17] demonstrated that laparoscopy was an independent predictor of time to postoperative chemotherapy by 25 days (50.1 days [laparoscopic] vs 75.2 days [open], P<.0001) due to the early recovery afforded by this approach. This outcome measure may be a more valuable measure of short-term benefit by its potential to translate into long-term oncologic advantage.

FUNCTIONAL OUTCOMES

Multiple trials have reported comparable rates of male and female sexual dysfunction following open or laparoscopic resection of rectal cancer.[18] In the CLASICC trial, overall sexual function was worse with laparoscopy owing to higher rates of TME in the laparoscopic group (80% vs 62% open), which was an independent predictor of male sexual dysfunction on multivariate analysis.[19] Comparison of patient-reported genitourinary function from the COLOR II trial found no difference in erectile dysfunction or micturition symptoms between the laparoscopic and open groups. Both cohorts had substantial worsening of sexual function after surgery, with partial recovery of function by 1 year. Bladder function was less affected than sexual function and recovered within 6 months. The functional assessment group represented only 62.7% of the original cohort with lower rates of leak and radiotherapy compared with nonrespondents, suggesting that these rates may underestimate the incidence of dysfunction.[20] The COREAN trial reported better physical functioning; less fatigue; and fewer micturition, gastrointestinal, and defecatory problems with laparoscopic resection. Short-term and long-term sexual function was similar between groups.[11]

ROBOTIC PROCTECTOMY

Robotic proctectomy addresses the problem of access to the deep pelvis with articulating instruments that improve retraction and maneuverability in the pelvis compared with rigid in-line laparoscopic instruments. The relative comfort of the robotic console also results in less surgeon fatigue compared with laparoscopy.[21] The technical advantage of the robotic platform is supported by a low rate of conversion and acceptable pathologic outcomes compared with laparoscopy. In review of the National Cancer Database comparing laparoscopic resection (n = 5447) versus robotic resection (n = 956), conversion was 9.5% (robotic) versus 16.4% (laparoscopic), with similar margin status and 30-day outcomes.[22] Baik and colleagues[23] support these findings along with shorter length of hospital stay of 5.7 days (robotic) versus

7.6 days (laparoscopic). In a randomized controlled trial of 163 patients by Kim and colleagues,[24] the rate of acceptable TME was high across groups (98.5% robotic vs 100% laparoscopic). Postoperative quality-of-life scoring was also similar with sexual function at 12 months favoring robotic resection.

The oncologic efficacy of robotic proctectomy is also supported by single-institution studies; Saklani and colleagues[25] report 3-year local recurrence of 2.7% robotic versus 6.3% laparoscopic ($P = .420$), with comparable rates of 3-year DFS and OS. Among patients undergoing ultralow TME at the same institution, Baek and colleagues[26] report equivalent postoperative outcomes, 3-year local recurrence, OS, and DFS between robotic and laparoscopic resection.

ROBOTIC OR LAPAROSCOPIC ANTERIOR RECTAL RESECTION TRIAL

The Robotic or Laparoscopic Anterior Rectal Resection trial (ROLARR) was conducted by 40 surgeons at 29 sites across 10 countries, randomizing 471 patients to receive robotic or laparoscopic resection for potentially curable rectal cancer. The primary endpoint was conversion rate, with additional oncologic, safety, and quality-of-life secondary endpoints. Only 24% of cancers were located in the low rectum. Robotic procedures were 37 minutes longer, on average, than laparoscopic procedures. The conversion rate was not significantly different (12.2% for laparoscopy vs 8.1% for robotic). CRM positivity and completeness of TME were also equivocal. Post hoc subset analysis identified obesity as a risk factor for conversion in the laparoscopic group only, suggesting that robotic surgery may offer an advantage in the obese pelvis.[27] A similar trial, COLRAR (Trial to Assess Robot-assisted Surgery and Laparoscopy-assisted Surgery in Patients With Mid or Low Rectal Cancer), is currently accruing patients in Korea with a primary endpoint of surgical quality as measured by TME and CRM positivity.[28]

TRANSANAL TOTAL MESORECTAL EXCISION

The past decade has seen renewed interest in an older surgical technique to address the technical challenges of access to the low pelvis. The transanal-transabdominal approach was introduced by Marks and colleagues[29,30] in the 1980s, offering transanal endoscopic micro-surgery–based resection of ultralow tumors with hand-sewn coloanal anastomosis for sphincter preservation. The technique has been modified to use the transanal minimally invasive surgery platform with standard laparoscopic equipment to provide better visualization and greater flexibility in surgical technique.[31] The combined transanal and transabdominal approach to produce a transanal TME (taTME) is an emerging technique.

Guiding principles of the taTME include transanal placement of a gas-tight pursestring suture in the anal canal above the intended distal margin of resection. Rectal division begins distal to the pursestring until the mesorectal plane (Heald's "holy plane") is entered. Circumferential mobilization of the mesorectum is carried cephalad until meeting the abdominal dissection around the level of the peritoneal reflection. Transabdominal resection is performed with a laparoscopic approach, although robotic-assisted transabdominal resection is also described.[32] Transanal dissection can precede, follow, or occur in concert with transabdominal dissection depending on institutional resources. TaTME promises an advantage for low or ultralow rectal cancers, distorted anatomy secondary to neoadjuvant therapy, the narrow male pelvis, significant visceral obesity (BMI>30), and in cases of prostatic hypertrophy.[33]

The ETAP-GRECCAR 11 Trial is a multicenter randomized controlled trial currently under way that is designed to evaluate the efficacy of taTME against laparoscopic TME.[34] Similarly, the COLOR III trial is an international multicenter randomized controlled trial currently in accrual, comparing taTME against laparoscopic TME with the primary endpoint of positive CRM. It is the hope that taTME will afford lower rates of CRM positivity and enable sphincter preservation particularly for low and mid rectal lesions.[35]

NATIONAL ACCREDITATION PROGRAM FOR RECTAL CANCER

Performance of a complete TME is a critical element in the optimal care of the patient with rectal cancer. Other essential elements include high-quality imaging to accurately stage the cancer before treatment, thorough pathologic evaluation of resection specimens, consistent adherence to adjuvant therapy guidelines, and a multidisciplinary team approach to treatment planning and quality improvement.[36,37] There is a great degree of variation in the quality of rectal cancer care provided in the United States. Many European countries have demonstrated improved outcomes after developing specialized centers for the treatment of rectal cancer.[38] The National Accreditation Program for Rectal Cancer (NAPRC) is a program of the American College of Surgeons and the Commission on Cancer that emphasizes a multidisciplinary, evidence-based approach to guide the processes of rectal cancer care and advocate for specialized centers to perform these high-risk procedures. The standards for accreditation arose from the work of the OSTRiCh (Optimizing the Surgical Treatment of Rectal Cancer) Consortium, an independent multispecialty collaborative dedicated to improving the quality of rectal cancer care in the United States by using the principles demonstrated to be effective in Europe.[39]

The absolute number of cases needed to optimize surgical outcomes remains unclear. Historically, high-volume surgeons (>20 cases) had fewer complications and need for postprocedural interventions compared with lower volume surgeons.[40] A more recent database analysis supports that surgeons with a cumulative 5-year experience of more than 25 rectal resections had significantly lower rates of major events (OR 0.82) and surgical complications (OR 0.71).[41] There are very few reports on the learning curve for laparoscopic resection of the rectum. The Z6051 trial required that surgeons be credentialed for laparoscopic and open TME rectal resection by submitting operative and pathology reports for 20 TME procedures, in addition to an unedited recording of a laparoscopic pelvic dissection for review. ROLARR required surgeons to have experience with at least 30 rectal cancer resections before credentialing. Certainly the excellent results reported in recent literature have become the expectation for clinical practice and colorectal surgeons who intend to manage rectal cancer should therefore undergo the same degree of scrutiny.

SUMMARY

TME can be safely performed through a minimally invasive approach by experienced surgeons and may offer patients benefit in certain short-term outcomes. Controversy remains regarding the optimal approach to TME for cancers in the low rectum. Long-term oncologic outcomes and meta-analysis of the most recent randomized controlled trials may offer additional clarity regarding the role of laparoscopic TME and those patients for whom the approach is most appropriate. Until then, laparoscopic TME should be used judiciously.

Emerging technologies, including robotic surgery and taTME, offer potential, but as yet are unproven alternative strategies for achieving the goal of a high-quality oncologic resection. As the landscape of rectal cancer surgery evolves, the necessary constant needs to be multidisciplinary oversight of rectal cancer surgery performed by surgeons and surgical centers experienced in this critically important procedure.

REFERENCES

1. Nelson H, Sargent DJ, Wieand HS, et al. A comparison of laparoscopically assisted and open colectomy for colon cancer. N Engl J Med 2004;350:2050–9.
2. Heald RJ, Husband EM, Ryall RD. The mesorectum in rectal cancer surgery—the clue to pelvic recurrence? Br J Surg 1982;69(10):613–6.
3. Quirke P, Durdey P, Dixon MF, et al. Local recurrence of rectal adenocarcinoma due to inadequate surgical resection: histopathological study of lateral tumour spread and surgical excision. Lancet 1986;2:996–9.
4. Martling AL, Holm T, Rutqvist LE. Effect of a surgical training programme on outcome of rectal cancer in the County of Stockholm. Lancet 2000;356:93–6.
5. MacFarlane JK, Ryall RDH, Heald RJ. Mesorectal excision for rectal cancer. Lancet 1993;341:457–60.
6. Fleshman JW, Wexner SD, Anvari M, et al. Laparoscopic vs. open abdominoperineal resection for cancer. Dis Colon Rectum 1999;42(7):930–9.
7. Feliciotti F, Guerrieri M, Paganini AM, et al. Long-term results of laparoscopic versus open resections for rectal cancer for 124 unselected patients. Surg Endosc 2003;17(10):1530–5.
8. Vennix S, Pelzers L, Bouvy N, et al. Laparoscopic versus open total mesorectal excision for rectal cancer. Cochrane Database Syst Rev 2014;58(4):CD005200.
9. Guillou PJ, Quirke P, Thorpe H, et al. Short-term endpoints of conventional versus laparoscopic-assisted surgery in patients with colorectal cancer (MRC CLASICC trial): multicentre, randomised controlled trial. Lancet 2005;365:1718–26.
10. Green BL, Marshall HC, Collinson F, et al. Long-term follow-up of the Medical Research Council CLASICC trial of conventional versus laparoscopically assisted resection in colorectal cancer. Br J Surg 2012;100(1):75–82.
11. Kang S-B, Park JW, Jeong S-Y, et al. Open versus laparoscopic surgery for mid or low rectal cancer after neoadjuvant chemoradiotherapy (COREAN trial): short-term outcomes of an open-label randomised controlled trial. Lancet Oncol 2010; 11(7):637–45.
12. Jeong S-Y, Park JW, Nam BH, et al. Open versus laparoscopic surgery for mid-rectal or low-rectal cancer after neoadjuvant chemoradiotherapy (COREAN trial): survival outcomes of an open-label, non-inferiority, randomised controlled trial. Lancet Oncol 2014;15(7):767–74.
13. Bonjer HJ, Deijen CL, Abis GA, et al. A randomized trial of laparoscopic versus open surgery for rectal cancer. N Engl J Med 2015;372(14):1324–32.
14. Fleshman J, Branda M, Sargent DJ, et al. Effect of laparoscopic-assisted resection vs open resection of stage II or III rectal cancer on pathologic outcomes. JAMA 2015;314(13):1346–55.
15. Stevenson ARL, Solomon MJ, Lumley JW, et al. Effect of laparoscopic-assisted resection vs open resection on pathological outcomes in rectal cancer. JAMA 2015;314(13):1356–63.
16. Zheng J, Feng X, Yang Z, et al. The comprehensive therapeutic effects of rectal surgery are better in laparoscopy: a systematic review and meta-analysis. Oncotarget 2017;8(8):12717–29.
17. Strouch MJ, Zhou G, Fleshman JW, et al. Time to initiation of postoperative chemotherapy. Dis Colon Rectum 2013;56(8):945–51.
18. Celentano V, Cohen R, Warusavitarne J, et al. Sexual dysfunction following rectal cancer surgery. Int J Colorectal Dis 2017;32(11):1523–30.

19. Jayne DG, Brown JM, Thorpe H, et al. Bladder and sexual function following resection for rectal cancer in a randomized clinical trial of laparoscopic versus open technique. Br J Surg 2005;92(9):1124–32.

20. Andersson J, Abis G, Gellerstedt M, et al. Patient-reported genitourinary dysfunction after laparoscopic and open rectal cancer surgery in a randomized trial (CO-LOR II). Br J Surg 2014;101(10):1272–9.

21. Pigazzi A, Ellenhorn JDI, Ballantyne GH, et al. Robotic-assisted laparoscopic low anterior resection with total mesorectal excision for rectal cancer. Surg Endosc 2006;20(10):1521–5.

22. Speicher PJ, Englum BR, Ganapathi AM, et al. Robotic low anterior resection for rectal cancer. Ann Surg 2015;262(6):1040–5.

23. Baik SH, Kwon HY, Kim JS, et al. Robotic versus laparoscopic low anterior resection of rectal cancer: short-term outcome of a prospective comparative study. Ann Surg Oncol 2009;16(6):1480–7.

24. Kim MJ, Park SC, Park JW, et al. Robot-assisted versus laparoscopic surgery for rectal cancer: a phase II open label prospective randomized controlled trial. Ann Surg 2018;267(2):243–51.

25. Saklani AP, Lim DR, Hur H, et al. Robotic versus laparoscopic surgery for mid–low rectal cancer after neoadjuvant chemoradiation therapy: comparison of oncologic outcomes. Int J Colorectal Dis 2013;28(12):1689–98.

26. Baek SJ, AL-Asari S, Jeong DH, et al. Robotic versus laparoscopic coloanal anastomosis with or without intersphincteric resection for rectal cancer. Surg Endosc 2013;27(11):4157–63.

27. Collinson FJ, Jayne DG, Pigazzi A, et al. An international, multicentre, prospective, randomised, controlled, unblinded, parallel-group trial of robotic-assisted versus standard laparoscopic surgery for the curative treatment of rectal cancer. Int J Colorectal Dis 2011;27(2):233–41.

28. COLRAR. Available at: https://clinicaltrials.gov/ct2/show/NCT01423214. Accessed December 18, 2018.

29. Marks G, Mohiuddin M, Goldstein SD. Sphincter preservation for cancer of the distal rectum using high dose preoperative radiation. Int J Radiat Oncol Biol Phys 1988;15(5):1065–8.

30. Marks JH, Frenkel JL, D'Andrea AP, et al. Maximizing rectal cancer results: TEM and TATA techniques to expand sphincter preservation. Surg Oncol Clin N Am 2011;20(3):501–20, viii–ix.

31. Atallah S, Albert M, Larach S. Transanal minimally invasive surgery: a giant leap forward. Surg Endosc 2010;24(9):2200–5.

32. Bravo R, Trépanier JS, Arroyave MC, et al. Combined transanal total mesorectal excision (taTME) with laparoscopic instruments and abdominal robotic surgery in rectal cancer. Tech Coloproctol 2017;21(3):233–5.

33. Motson RW, Whiteford MH, Hompes R, et al. Current status of trans-anal total mesorectal excision (TaTME) following the Second International Consensus Conference. Colorectal Dis 2016;18(1):13–8.

34. Lelong B, de Chaisemartin C, Meillat H, et al. A multicentre randomised controlled trial to evaluate the efficacy, morbidity and functional outcome of endoscopic transanal proctectomy versus laparoscopic proctectomy for low-lying rectal cancer (ETAP-GRECCAR 11 TRIAL): rationale and design. BMC Cancer 2017;17:253.

35. COLOR III. Available at: https://clinicaltrials.gov/ct2/show/NCT02736942. Accessed December 18, 2018.

36. Dietz DW, Consortium for Optimizing Surgical Treatment of Rectal Cancer. Multidisciplinary management of rectal cancer: the OSTRICH. J Gastrointest Surg 2013;17:1863–8.

37. Abbas MA, Chang GJ, Read TE, et al. Optimizing rectal cancer management: analysis of current evidence. Dis Colon Rectum 2014;57:252–9.

38. Monson JRT, Probst CP, Wexner SD, et al. Failure of evidence-based cancer care in the United States. Ann Surg 2014;260:625–32.

39. NAPRC. Available at: https://www.facs.org/quality-programs/cancer/naprc. Accessed December 18, 2018.

40. Billingsley KG, Morris AM, Green P, et al. Does surgeon case volume influence nonfatal adverse outcomes after rectal cancer resection? J Am Coll Surg 2008; 206(6):1167–77.

41. Yeo HL, Abelson JS, Mao J, et al. Surgeon annual and cumulative volumes predict early postoperative outcomes after rectal cancer resection. Ann Surg 2017; 265(1):151–7.

Minimally Invasive Surgery for Primary and Metastatic Adrenal Malignancy

Colleen M. Kiernan, MD, MPH*, Jeffrey E. Lee, MD

KEYWORDS

- Adrenalectomy • Adrenocortical carcinoma • Adrenal metastasis • Laparoscopic
- Minimally invasive • Retroperitoneoscopic

KEY POINTS

- Adrenal lesions suspicious for malignancy warrant thoughtful consideration of the patient's history, physical, biochemical, and imaging evaluation when determining the preferred operative approach.
- Minimally invasive adrenalectomy is the preferred surgical approach in selected patients with isolated, moderately sized metastatic disease to the adrenal gland, a good performance status, and otherwise favorable tumor biology.
- Localized, moderately sized adrenal lesions potentially representing a primary malignancy may be considered for a minimally invasive approach by surgeons experienced in the technique.
- Minimally invasive adrenalectomy for primary adrenal malignancy should be avoided because of the likelihood that intraoperative direct manipulation of the typically friable tumor will lead to tumor capsular disruption, fragmentation, and/or incomplete resection, with an associated increased risk of local-regional recurrence and peritoneal carcinomatosis.

INTRODUCTION

Minimally invasive adrenal surgery (MIS) was first described by Gagner in 1992, when he reported successful MIS extirpation of the adrenal gland in 3 patients with functional adrenal tumors. He proposed that the resultant decreased length of hospital stay and postoperative pain observed with the utilization of MIS would make this approach particularly helpful in the surgical management of asymptomatic adrenal lesions.[1]

Disclosure Statement: The authors have no financial disclosures.
Department of Surgical Oncology, MD Anderson Cancer Center, 1515 Holcombe Boulevard, Houston, TX 77030, USA
* Corresponding author.
E-mail address: CMKiernan@mdanderson.org

Surg Oncol Clin N Am 28 (2019) 309–326
https://doi.org/10.1016/j.soc.2018.11.011
1055-3207/19/© 2018 Elsevier Inc. All rights reserved.

Over the past 25 years, MIS adrenalectomy has become the preferred approach for most of the patients with adrenal tumors, including but not limited to benign nonfunctioning tumors, benign functional tumors, selected metastases to the adrenal gland, and select indeterminate adrenal nodules (largely benign adrenal cortical adenomas). The benefits of MIS include decreased blood loss, transfusion requirement, procedure times, hospital stay, and complications when compared with open adrenalectomy.[2–7]

However, MIS adrenalectomy for primary adrenal malignancy (ie, adrenocortical carcinoma [ACC]) remains controversial due to the uncertainty regarding oncologic outcomes relative to open adrenalectomy.[8–11]

In this article, the authors discuss the evaluation of adrenal nodules concerning for malignancy and review the indications for MIS adrenalectomy in adrenal nodules suspicious for malignancy. They also describe important patient and tumor factors to consider when making the decision to proceed with MIS adrenalectomy. The current literature on MIS adrenal metastasectomy and its association with survival by tumor type are also reviewed. The authors also discuss the available data and current recommendations regarding MIS adrenalectomy for ACC.

CONTENT
Evaluation of Adrenal Nodules Concerning for Malignancy

In the last 2 decades, the number of adrenalectomies performed in the United States has increased.[12,13] The cause of this increase is likely multifactorial and includes increased frequency of performance and improved quality of cross-sectional abdominal imaging, which has resulted in increased frequency of identification of adrenal "incidentalomas" (defined as an asymptomatic adrenal nodule discovered in a patient for whom the imaging study was performed for an unrelated reason) as well as the likely identification of an increased number of functioning adrenal nodules with relatively milder associated symptoms (eg, "subclinical" Cushing syndrome, aldosteronomas, pheochromocytomas). Although most of this increase in identification of adrenal nodules has been of benign adrenal tumors, the rate of adrenalectomy and more specifically MIS adrenalectomy for malignancy is also increasing.[12–14]

The most common indications for MIS adrenalectomy are summarized in **Box 1**. For the purposes of the current discussion, the authors focus on adrenal masses that are concerning for, or are known to represent, primary or metastatic cancer.

Box 1
Potential indications for adrenalectomy

Nonfunctioning adrenal nodules

Functional adrenal tumors

  Pheochromocytoma

  Cushing syndrome

  Cushing disease

  Aldosteronomas

  Virilizing tumors

Myelolipoma

Adrenocortical carcinoma

Metastasis to the adrenal gland

As described in American Association of Clinical Endocrinologists and American Association of Endocrine Surgeons Medical Guidelines for the Management of Adrenal Incidentalomas, in the evaluation of any adrenal lesion there are 3 essential questions to address: (1) Is the tumor functional (has it resulted in circulating hormone excess)? (2) Does the tumor have radiographic features concerning for malignancy? (3) Does the patient have a history of malignancy, and is it therefore possible that the adrenal tumor represents metastatic cancer?[15]

The following sections review the recommended clinical, biochemical, and imaging evaluation of adrenal tumors suspicious for malignancy.

Clinical evaluation

A detailed history and physical focusing on signs and symptoms associated with functional adrenal tumors including signs and symptoms of hypercortisolism (weight gain, central obesity, easy bruisability, peripheral muscle wasting, hypertension, diabetes, virilization), hyperaldosteronism (hypertension, fluid retention, history of hypokalemia, muscle cramping, weakness), and pheochromocytoma (hypertension, headache, weight loss, anxiety, sweating, palpitation, or history of arrhythmia). The history should also include relevant personal risk factors (sun exposure, smoking) and family history of malignancy (including history that suggests multiple endocrine neoplasia (MEN) and/or von Hippel-Lindau syndrome) as well as a history of surveillance colonoscopy and mammogram and/or dermatologic examination for pigmented lesions. Inquiry into systemic symptoms such as weight loss, fatigue, anorexia, or back pain should also be performed, because these suggest either an advanced cancer process or, in the case of bilateral adrenal involvement by metastasis, adrenal insufficiency.

Biochemical evaluation

Recommended initial screening tests and their positive results are summarized in **Table 1**.

The goal of screening biochemical evaluation is to assess for the likely presence of hypercortisolism, hyperaldosteronism, or catecholamine excess. This evaluation is essential even when a malignant primary or metastatic lesion is suspected, because identification of a functional mass will affect management, and functioning adrenal cortical and medullary tumors are predicted to occur incidentally in patients with a history of cancer at least as commonly as in those without such a history. Screening for hormone over-production can optionally be skipped in patients who are referred with a

Table 1
Initial biochemical evaluation of an adrenal mass

	Screening Test	Positive Result—Warrants Further Evaluation
Hypercortisolism	Overnight 1 mg dexamethasone suppression test	Serum cortisol >5 ug/dL with suppressed ACTH
Hyperaldosteronism	Plasma aldosterone, plasma renin	Ratio of plasma aldosterone concentration to plasma renin activity >20
Pheochromocytoma	Plasma free metanephrine and normetanephrine levels and/or 24 h urine metanephrines	Plasma metanephrines >3–4x normal or 24 h total urine metanephrine > 1800ug

Abbreviation: ACTH, adrenocorticotropic hormone.
Data from Zeiger MA, Thompson GB, Duh QY, et al. American Association of Clinical Endocrinologists and American Association of Endocrine Surgeons Medical guidelines for the management of adrenal incidentalomas: executive summary of recommendations. Endocr Pract 2009;15(5):450–3.

biopsy-proven metastasis to the adrenal gland; however, patients with bilateral adrenal tumors suspected of representing bilateral adrenal metastases from a known or unknown primary site should undergo cortisol and adrenocorticotropic hormone (ACTH) determination to screen for the presence of occult adrenal insufficiency.

Approximately two-thirds of ACCs produce and release excess hormones, and known hormone hypersecretion can affect perioperative management, prognosis, and treatment of recurrent and metastatic disease and therefore should be evaluated preoperatively.[16,17]

In addition, the reported rate of adrenal metastases in patients with a prior history of cancer who present with an adrenal mass is 27% to 73%.[18,19] Thus not all adrenal masses in patients with a prior history of malignancy will be metastatic disease; they can represent functional or nonfunctional benign adenomas or pheochromocytomas. Therefore, before performing a biopsy of an adrenal lesion concerning for metastasis, biochemical evaluation for pheochromocytoma is recommended to obviate the risk of hypertensive crisis.[20,21]

Radiographic features concerning for malignancy

The 2 most commonly used imaging modalities in the initial evaluation of patients with adrenal tumors are computerized tomography (CT) scan and MRI. In general, malignant adrenal lesions are heterogeneous in appearance with an irregular shape and indistinct margins. ACCs tend to be large (>6 cm) and exhibit rapid growth; in contrast, metastatic lesions can present at a range of different sizes and exhibit variable growth patterns.[22] **Box 2** summarizes radiographic features concerning for malignancy.

The imaging evaluation of an adrenal mass typically includes precontrast images, contrast images in both arterial and portal venous phases, as well as delayed imaging 10 to 15 minutes after contrast administration. However, if initial noncontrast imaging demonstrates an adrenal mass with Hounsfield unit (HU) density less than 10, further contrast and delayed imaging is not considered necessary due to the high specificity (98%) of that finding in predicting a lipid-rich benign cortical adenoma.[23,24] In practice, pre- and postcontrast images are usually obtained sequentially as a routine within part of the same, standardized imaging protocol.

Approximately 30% of adrenal masses have an indeterminate precontrast HU (ie, between 10 and 30), thus justifying contrast-enhanced CT with delayed washout.[25] Primary and metastatic malignant adrenal tumors tend to have increased and persistent

---

Box 2
Imaging features concerning for malignancy

Imaging Features Concerning for Potential Adrenal Malignancy

Size >4 cm

Growth in size >1 cm on serial imaging (within 1 year)

Irregular shape

Heterogeneous

Poorly defined margins

Necrosis

Hounsfield unit >10 on noncontrasted imaging

<60% washout on CT imaging

Hyperintense on MRI T2-weighted imaging

contrast accumulation due to neovascularization of the tumor and therefore demonstrate less washout of contrast on delayed imaging (**Fig. 1**). Thus, calculating the absolute or relative washout of indeterminate lesions can be helpful in further characterizing the lesion. Contrast washout can be calculated in 2 ways: absolute percentage washout (APW), calculated by dividing the values of enhanced HU minus the delayed HU by the value of the enhanced HU minus the noncontract HU multiplied by 100; or relative percentage washout (RPW), calculated based on an initial CT scan with contrast and delayed scans only by diving the value of the enhanced HU minus the delayed HU by the enhanced HU multiplied by 100. An APW greater than 60% or an RPW greater than 40% is consistent with a benign adenoma (APW sensitivity 56%–100% and specificity 98%–100%; RPW sensitivity 82% and specificity 92%).[26–28]

In summary, CT findings of precontrast density greater than 10 HU and less than 60% absolute washout are features concerning for malignancy. However, these findings can also be seen in pheochromocytomas, and it is emphasized also that so-called "atypical" lipid-poor but benign adrenocortical adenomas can exhibit similar imaging characteristics (eg, precontrast HU between 10 and 30), and thus imaging alone may not be diagnostic.

Because of its outstanding spatial resolution, CT is also helpful in providing the surgeon with information regarding local invasion, the presence of bilateral or multifocal primary tumors (eg, in patients with an inherited pheochromocytoma syndrome) and the presence of extraadrenal metastatic disease (in patients with primary adrenal malignancy or an extraadrenal malignancy metastatic to the adrenal gland).

MRI can also be helpful, particularly when iodinated contrast is contraindicated or avoidance of radiation exposure is desired. MRI can be particularly useful in identifying pheochromocytomas and in distinguishing among benign adenomas, malignant tumors, and pheochromocytomas. Adenomas typically exhibit low signal intensity on

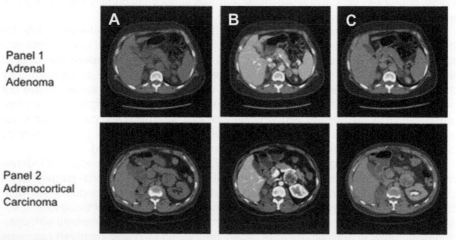

Panel 1
Adrenal
Adenoma

Panel 2
Adrenocortical
Carcinoma

Fig. 1. CT imaging of adrenal adenoma compared with adrenocortical carcinoma. Representative CT imaging of an adrenal adenoma and adrenocortical carcinoma in (*A*) precontrast imaging, (*B*) contrast imaging, and (*C*) 15-minute delayed imaging. Panel 1 demonstrates characteristic findings of an adrenal adenoma with low-density precontrast imaging and rapid washout of contrast on 15-minute delayed imaging. Panel 2 demonstrates a large, heterogeneous left adrenal mass with increased density of precontrasted imaging with increased arterial enhancement on contrasted imaging and incomplete washout on 15-minute delayed imaging in a patient with ACC.

both T1- and T2-weighted images; malignant lesions demonstrate enhancement on T2-weighted images; and pheochromocytomas are characteristically intensely enhancing on T2 imaging.[28] However, as with CT, there is overlap between the imaging characteristics of pheochromocytomas and benign primary and metastatic adrenal malignancies; therefore, adrenal MRI results must be interpreted with the patient's clinical history and biochemical evaluation in mind.

Role of biopsy for adrenal nodules concerning for malignancy Adrenal biopsy is generally recommended only in situations in which the results will influence management—for example, to confirm the presence of isolated metastasis to the adrenal gland in a patient with a history of malignancy at risk for adrenal metastasis in whom confirmation of the presence of metastatic cancer would result in a recommendation for systemic therapy. Adrenal biopsy should be avoided in lesions concerning for ACC, unless required to initiate systemic therapy (eg, a patient with borderline resectable or metastatic ACC).[29–32]

Before performing adrenal biopsy for suspected metastasis, biochemical evaluation for pheochromocytoma is recommended (eg, plasma fractionated metanephrines). The evaluation and management of patients with adrenal metastasis is discussed in subsequent sections.

Minimally Invasive Adrenalectomy for Indeterminate Adrenal Nodules Concerning for Malignancy

In this section, the authors review operative management of an indeterminate adrenal nodule concerning for malignancy.

An adrenal nodule can be considered indeterminate when it is intermediate in size (>4 cm but <6 cm) or has demonstrated greater than or equal to 1 cm growth in 1 year or less, has imaging characteristics that are not consistent with a benign adenoma, and/or has clinical or biochemical features suggesting primary malignancy (eg, virilization) (see **Box 2**).

The size cut-off recommendations for surgery of an incidental adrenal nodule are based on reported malignancy rates, with lesions less than or equal to 4 cm with malignancy rates of approximately 2% or less, 4.1 to 6 cm with malignancy rates of approximately 6%, and greater than 6 cm with malignancy rates of approximately 25%.[15,18] The rate of malignancy of lesions with combinations of indeterminate but suspicious characteristics is not well described, and therefore judgment is required when deciding on surgery and optimal surgical approach for patients with, for example, relatively small adrenal nodules with indeterminate imaging characteristics or those that demonstrate some degree of growth on serial imaging.

Several different surgical approaches have been proposed for resection of indeterminate adrenal nodules. There are clear advantages to MIS adrenal surgery when compared with open adrenalectomy in regard to acute perioperative outcomes. Multiple prospective and retrospective studies have demonstrated lower blood loss, operative times, hospital length of stay, and morbidity with MIS when compared with open adrenalectomy. In addition, patients report decreased pain and improved cosmesis with MIS adrenalectomy.[2–7]

The decision to approach these lesions using an MIS approach should be patient and surgeon specific. Surgeons should choose the approach they are most familiar with, have had sufficient training in, and have the best patient outcomes with.[33] Recent studies have shown that the median average annual volume for surgeons performing adrenalectomy is 1 case.[34,35] These same studies demonstrate improved outcomes when adrenalectomies are performed by high-volume surgeons (defined as 4–6 adrenalectomies annually). For surgeons experienced in both anterior transabdominal LA as well as posterior retroperitoneoscopic (PRA) approaches, and assuming the patient is eligible for either approach based on tumor type and anatomic considerations, recent randomized trial data suggest that both approaches are equally safe, with similar operative times, blood loss, postoperative levels of patient discomfort, and recovery times.[36,37] Therefore, the details of considerations provided in **Table 2** help guide the operative approach in such situations.

Patient factors may dictate the operative approach. Patients who have had previous transabdominal operations may benefit from PRA to avoid potential adhesive disease.[38–40] In addition, tumor size may affect the MIS approach chosen, because larger tumors (>6 cm or so) may be more challenging to extirpate via a retroperitoneal approach due to smaller working volume compared with the anterior transabdominal approach.[39–41] However, it is also emphasized that properly performed PRA of small-to medium-sized tumors generally allows for minimal need to directly manipulate or grasp the adrenal gland or the tumor, thus minimizing the risk of capsular disruption, and patient recovery is at least as rapid as reported for the anterior laparoscopic approach. Patient body habitus is also an important factor to consider, because morbidly obese patients with abundant intraabdominal and retroperitoneal fat will demonstrate compression of the retroperitoneal space from their intraabdominal organs secondary when in the prone position. Furthermore, such patients may have such a large distance between their skin and the retroperitoneal space at the site of PRA port placement (beneath the tip of the 12th rib) that standard- or obesity-length ports are simply not long enough to permit effective access.[40,41] In such patients, the increased working space provided by the laparoscopic transabdominal (LA) approach, the lateral positioning that allows for gravity to help move the intraabdominal contents away from the adrenal gland, and the common finding that subcutaneous fat distance is actually lower in the upper anterior abdomen than posteriorly just above the hips can all favor LA.

Each approach as well as its associated advantages and disadvantages are described in **Table 2**. No matter the approach, it is essential to respect oncologic principles in any lesion suspicious for malignancy. Thus, the tumor must be removed completely and intact. Thus, the MIS approach is considered preferable for lesions with atypical imaging features potentially representing primary malignancy but is more likely to be representative of an atypical benign lesion, for example, intermediate size, lack of intratumor fat, and growth on serial imaging. It is emphasized that in patients with clear evidence of primary ACC (adrenal tumor not suspected of representing a metastasis with necrosis, irregular borders, local invasion, or regional nodal involvement), it is far better to start open than to start MIS, encounter some combination of capsular disruption, fragmentation, or uncontrolled hemorrhage, and convert to open.[33]

Management of Adrenal Metastases

Isolated metastases to the adrenal gland most commonly originate from the lung; however, other common sites of primary malignancy include melanoma, kidney, colon, breast, and lymphoma.[42–47] Although prospective data are generally lacking, multiple retrospective investigations have demonstrated that adrenalectomy in highly selected patients with isolated or oligometastatic disease from primary sites including the lung, melanoma, and kidney can result in prolonged survival duration and improved survival compared with similar patients who do not undergo adrenalectomy.[42,44,45,47–50]

Metastasis to the adrenal gland should be considered in patients with an adrenal mass and a history of malignancy that has a tendency to spread to the adrenal.

Table 2
Commonly used minimally invasive adrenal surgery operative approaches to the adrenal gland

Operative Approach	Advantages	Disadvantages	Patient Factors to Consider
Laparoscopic Transabdominal Adrenalectomy (LA)	• Large working space • Familiar orientation of anatomy	• Requires mobilization of intraabdominal organs • Must reposition for bilateral adrenalectomy	• Useful in morbidly obese patients • May be difficult in patients with prior abdominal surgery
Posterior Retroperitoneoscopic Adrenalectomy (PRA)	• Direct access to gland • Avoids intraabdominal cavity • Single position for bilateral adrenalectomy	• Lack of access to abdomen for exploration or control of hemorrhage • Difficulty in removing large tumors • Can be difficult in obese patients • Decreased working space	• Distance from skin to gland in obese patients • Ability to tolerate prone positioning
Lateral Retroperitoneoscopic Adrenalectomy	• Familiar approach to the gland for surgeons who routinely perform laparoscopic nephrectomy • Avoids the intraabdominal cavity	• Difficulty in removing large tumors • Requires more ports than LA or PRA	
Robotic Adrenalectomy (LA or PRA)	• Useful in patients with high BMI • Can be used for larger tumors (>5.5 cm) • 3-dimensional depth perception, additional dexterity	• Cost • Learning curve • Complexity	• Similar to patient factors to consider for LA or PRA

Abbreviation: BMI, body mass index.

Evaluation in such patients should include imaging with abdominal CT or MRI, which should be compared with prior abdominal imaging. In addition, biochemical evaluation for a functional adrenal tumor should be pursued (see prior sections on biochemical evaluation and imaging).

If metastatic disease is suspected based on history, imaging, and biochemical evaluation, the patient should undergo evaluation for extraadrenal disease. The evaluation required will vary by primary tumor type but may include, for example, whole body PET/CT, dedicated chest CT, and/or MRI of the brain. The decision to proceed with adrenalectomy for metastatic cancer warrants thoughtful consideration of the natural history of the underlying disease, tumor biology, presence of extraadrenal disease (if any), patient performance status, and availability of alternative therapeutic options (eg, systemic or radiation therapy).[45]

Adrenal biopsy has been demonstrated to have high sensitivity, specificity, and negative predictive value for distinguishing benign from metastatic adrenal tumors (92%, 94%, and 100%, respectively).[51,52] Biopsy can be particularly helpful in patients with a new, isolated adrenal mass suspicious for metastasis in a patient with a prior relevant cancer when the biopsy would (1) establish the new onset of distant metastatic disease, (2) allow for initiation of systemic therapy, and/or (3) confirm eligibility of the patient for entry into a clinical trial. However, not every adrenal mass suspicious for adrenal metastasis requires biopsy. Newly identified or rapidly enlarging adrenal tumors not present on prior imaging in a patient with a history of a known malignancy with propensity to metastasize to the adrenal glands (eg, lung, melanoma, renal cell carcinoma) are highly likely to represent adrenal metastasis. In such patients, and in the absence of an attractive alternative systemic treatment option or following induction systemic therapy, a decision may be made to proceed directly to surgical resection without preoperative biopsy.

Oncologic benefits of adrenalectomy in metastatic disease
Several retrospective investigations have examined the outcomes of adrenalectomy for metastatic disease. One study used the Surveillance, Epidemiology, and End Results (SEER) database from 1992 to 2010 to match 166 patients who underwent adrenalectomy for adrenal metastases from kidney, lung, sarcoma, colon, pancreas, and other primary sites to similar patients who did not undergo adrenalectomy. This study found that patients with soft-tissue, kidney, lung, and pancreatic tumors had a better overall survival at 3 years with adrenalectomy: sarcoma (86% vs 30%), kidney (72% vs 27%), lung (52% vs 25%), and pancreas (45% vs 12%). In this cohort, they identified shorter interval from primary diagnosis to adrenalectomy, other distant sites of disease, surgery for palliation and persistent disease as risk factors for death.[50]

In a multicenter European study of 317 patients who underwent adrenalectomy for solid tumor metastases, the investigators found that patients with renal cell carcinoma, metachronous lesions, and isolated adrenal metastases had more favorable outcomes than patients with non–small cell lung cancer (NSCLC), colorectal cancer, or synchronous metastases. Patients with renal cell cancer who underwent adrenalectomy had a median survival of 84 months, NSCLC 26 months and colorectal cancer 29 months. Patients with metachronous adrenal metastases had a median survival of 30 months compared with 23 months for those with synchronous metastases. In this study, 46% of adrenalectomies were performed using an MIS approach, demonstrating the widespread application of this approach to patients with adrenal metastasis. Interestingly, their multivariate cox proportional hazards model, MIS adrenalectomy, was associated with a survival advantage with a hazard ratio of 0.65, 95% confidence interval 0.47 to 0.89, $P = -.009$.[44]

In a study of 154 patients with melanoma metastatic to the adrenal gland treated at the authors' institution (notably before the availability of the current generation of targeted and immune-based therapies), outcomes of patients who underwent adrenalectomy were compared with outcomes of those who did not undergo adrenalectomy. Twenty-two patients underwent surgery. Twenty patients were rendered disease free by adrenalectomy alone (n = 14) or adrenalectomy with concomitant extraadrenal metastasectomy (n = 6). Patients who underwent adrenalectomy had an improved overall survival compared with those managed nonoperatively (20.7 months vs 6.8 months, P<.001). This study suggests that metastatic melanoma isolated to the adrenal, normal lactate dehydrogenase, symptoms related to adrenal metastasis, a disease-free interval of 1 year or more, and limited extraadrenal disease that can also be resected may be reasonable selection criteria when considering to proceed with adrenalectomy, although this treatment paradigm should be updated in the era of modern melanoma systemic therapy.[49]

Operative approach to adrenal metastatic disease

Minimally invasive adrenalectomy has become the preferred operative approach for management of adrenal metastasis. It has been demonstrated to be both safe and oncologically appropriate in selected patients.[45,46,53–57] A retrospective review of 94 adrenalectomies for isolated adrenal metastases (63 open and 31 MIS) found no difference in local recurrence, margin status, disease free interval, or overall survival based on the surgical approach chosen. Moreover, MIS adrenalectomy was associated with decreased blood loss (106 vs 749 cc, P<.001), operative time (175 vs 208 mins, P = .04), length of stay (2.8 vs 8 days, P<.001), and complication rate (4% vs 34%, P<.01).[46]

However, other studies have suggested that for large tumors (>5–6 cm) MIS adrenalectomy is associated with increased risk of a margin-positive resection and an increased complication rate.[47] Therefore, when determining the operative approach to adrenal metastases, tumor size and radiographic evidence for local invasion should be considered. Finally, MIS adrenalectomy, particularly via a PRA approach, may limit the ability to evaluate and treat other intraabdominal sites of metastasis (eg, melanoma metastatic to the small intestine) and may therefore be relatively contraindicated in patients with known or suspected extraadrenal but intraabdominal sites of oligometastasis for which concomitant surgery would be desired.

Adrenocortical Carcinoma

ACC is a rare primary adrenal malignancy with an annual incidence of 1 to 2 per million.[58,59] It is an aggressive tumor that carries a poor prognosis. Most patients present with locally advanced or metastatic disease not amenable to surgical resection.

ACC is commonly diagnosed during evaluation of symptoms related to hormone excess because approximately two-thirds of ACCs produce and release excess hormones.[16,17] Up to one-third of patients will present with nonspecific symptoms due to tumor growth such as abdominal or flank pain, abdominal fullness, or early satiety or be found incidentally on imaging for unrelated medical issues.[60]

Biochemical evaluation should include screening for cortisol overproduction, pheochromocytoma, and aldosteronoma if hypertensive and/or hypokalemic. Sex hormones should be evaluated in anyone with virilizing features or imaging characteristics suspicious for ACC.

Imaging of an adrenal mass suspicious for ACC should include an adrenal protocol CT or MRI. On CT, ACC is typically identified as a large heterogeneous mass with indistinct borders. Invasion of adjacent structures is common, including liver, kidney, and vena cava on the right side and pancreas, spleen, renal vein, and kidney on the left side. Vena cava tumor thrombus is common, often originating at the level of the right adrenal vein and extending into the retrohepatic cava or extending from the left renal vein into the infrahepatic vena cava. Regional lymphadenopathy may also be seen. If ACC is suspected based on imaging, a CT of the chest should be performed to evaluate for pulmonary metastasis; pulmonary emboli are also common in patients with ACC.

Operative approach to adrenocortical carcinoma

Complete surgical resection with negative margins is the only curative option for ACC.[9,58,61–63] Thus the operative approach chosen must have the highest likelihood of achieving this goal. Controversy continues to exist on the role of an MIS approach in surgical management of primary ACC.

Proponents of the MIS approach to ACC cite retrospective series that conclude that an MIS approach is safe and can achieve similar oncologic outcomes for highly selected patients with relatively "small" tumors (<10 cm) without evidence of local invasion, provided oncologic principals are respected.[64–68] In contrast, proponents of open adrenalectomy cite retrospective studies of referral populations of patients with ACC that have identified increased rates of peritoneal carcinomatosis, capsular disruption, positive margins, and recurrence, as well as poorer stage-specific survival, in patients undergoing MIS compared with open resection of primary ACC.[9–11] There are no randomized controlled studies comparing MIS to open adrenalectomy for ACC and almost certainly never will be due to the rare nature of the disease and other considerations.

The American Association of Clinical Endocrinologists/American Association of Endocrine Surgeons, the Society of American Gastrointestinal and Endoscopic Surgeons, as well as the European Network for the Study of Adrenal Tumors guidelines all agree that open adrenalectomy should be performed if ACC is suspected.[15,33,69]

ACC is often a soft tumor with consistency similar to friable adrenal cortex; capsular disruption and fragmentation are easy to induce, particularly during direct tumor manipulation that commonly occurs in attempted MIS of these characteristically large tumors. Furthermore, ACC tends to invade through the tumor capsule with microscopic disease present at the gland surface; thus minimizing direct contact with the tumor surface is essential to avoid violating the tumor capsule or causing disruption of disease at the surface of the gland.[58] Thus, the authors endorse with the aforementioned consensus guidelines favoring open adrenalectomy for ACC, because the open approach they believe maximizes the likelihood of complete en bloc resection of an intact tumor and facilitates an appropriate regional operation, including any indicated lymphadenectomy.

The role of lymph node dissection in treatment of ACC remains unclear; there is no consensus regarding the extent of lymph node dissection that should be routinely performed, if any. Reported rates of lymph node removal in studies using large national databases are low (17%–30%).[16,70,71] Standardization of regional lymphadenectomy has been proposed to include first-order drainage nodes including the renal hilum lymph nodes, celiac lymph nodes, and the paraaortic and paracaval lymph nodes above the renal pedicle and ipsilateral to the adrenal gland.[72] However, this definition has not been widely adopted. A study of the German ACC Registry reports that in 283 patients with ACC formal lymph node dissection based on adrenal lymphatic drainage patterns results in a reduced risk of tumor recurrence (hazard ratio [HR] = 0.65, $P = .42$) and disease-related death (HR = 0.54, $P = .049$).[71] The rate of lymph node dissection is lower in adrenalectomies performed using an MIS approach for ACC than in those performed open.[73] Important missing data in these retrospective series is the proportion of patients who underwent lymph node removal of involved regional nodes for preoperatively or intraoperatively defined indications rather than routinely (that is, because of the presence of suspicious nodes identified either on preoperative imaging or intraoperatively, or because the involved nodes were within the field of adjacent organ resection, eg, pancreas, spleen, or kidney). The authors' current practice is to resect lymph nodes based on these latter criteria rather than performing routine lymphadenectomy.

Patients with primary ACC can present with formally resectable tumors, but with characteristics arguing against immediate surgery, including an unacceptably high risk for incomplete resection or early recurrence or an unacceptably high risk of perioperative morbidity or mortality. Such characteristics included a large and extensive primary tumor and need for multiorgan resection (liver, pancreas, kidney), significant vena cava tumor thrombus, documented or suspected oligometastatic disease, and potentially correctable comorbidities (severe Cushing syndrome, pulmonary emboli). Such patients may be considered to have borderline resectable ACC and be candidates for preoperative (neoadjuvant) systemic therapy. Early experience suggests such an approach, combined with appropriately aggressive surgical resection, can result in good outcomes compared with patients treated with upfront open surgery.[29]

Finally, the importance of surgeon experience in resection of ACC cannot be underemphasized due to the often-complex nature of these tumors. Lack of experience with adrenal tumors can lead to tumor rupture and/or positive margins regardless of approach. Several studies have demonstrated higher rates of complete resection and improved outcomes when ACCs are managed at centers with expertise.[62,68,74–76] In this context it is important to emphasize that in the United States 45% of adrenalectomies for ACC are performed in community hospitals, 30% in academic centers, and only 15% in National Cancer Institute–designated Cancer Centers.[70] Referral to high-volume centers, experienced in treating patients with ACC, should be considered before proceeding with resection, regardless of operative approach.

CLINICAL EXAMPLES AND MANAGEMENT

Patient 1: a 43-year-old woman presented with chronic back and abdominal pain. She had a CT scan performed 5 years ago that demonstrated a 2.7 cm L adrenal nodule. She had no signs or symptoms of hormone hypersecretion. She had no previous history of malignancy. A CT scan performed during current evaluation demonstrated a 4.4 cm left adrenal nodule (**Fig. 2**). Biochemical evaluation included baseline AM cortisol of 9.6 ug/dL and ACTH of 6 pg/mL. A 1 mg overnight dexamethasone test failed to suppress her AM cortisol level. Her plasma metanephrines were normal. She was diagnosed with subclinical Cushing syndrome. Although increasing in size, the mass had the appearance of a benign adrenal adenoma on imaging. She was therefore recommended to undergo MIS via PRA. Pathology revealed a benign adrenal adenoma.

Patient 2: a 67-year-old man presented with metastatic melanoma from an unknown primary site to the subcutaneous tissue, lung, bone, gastrointestinal tract, and left adrenal gland. He received immune checkpoint inhibitor and subsequently demonstrated complete response at all sites except for the left adrenal gland. His body mass index is 39, and on review of imaging he was thought to be of borderline habitus for PRA due to increased distance between the skin and retroperitoneal space (see **Fig. 2**). He therefore underwent MIS via an anterior LA. Pathology was consistent with treated melanoma, with no viable tumor cells present.

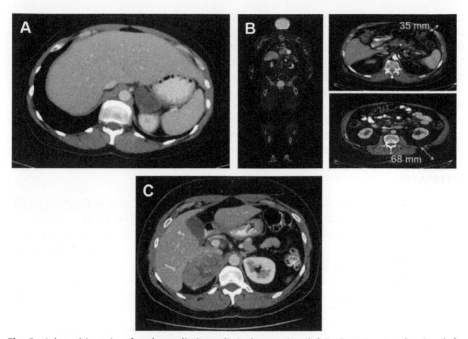

Fig. 2. Adrenal imaging for three distinct clinical scenarios. (*A*) Patient 1: an enlarging left adrenal mass. This abdominal CT demonstrates a 4.4 cm left adrenal mass that is low density and relatively homogenous, without evidence of local invasion of surrounding structures. (*B*) Patient 2: metastatic melanoma to left adrenal gland in a patient with a body mass index of 39. The PET CT demonstrates a single PET-avid lesion in left adrenal gland consistent with isolated melanoma metastasis. Abdominal CT localizes the left adrenal mass and also allows for measurement of the distance from the skin to the retroperitoneal space to assist in operative planning. Because of the large skin-to-retroperitoneal distance beneath the tip of the left 12th rib and the smaller skin-to-peritoneal distance in the left upper abdomen, LA rather than PRA was performed. (*C*) Patient 3: patient with a symptomatic adrenal mass representing ACC. This abdominal CT demonstrates a 9 cm right adrenal mass that is heterogeneous and irregular and is therefore concerning for ACC.

Patient 3: a 51-year-old woman presented with hypertension and hirsutism. A CT scan was performed for abdominal pain suspected of representing diverticulitis. A 9 cm right adrenal mass was identified. The mass was heterogeneous and irregular (see **Fig. 2**). Biochemical evaluation revealed elevated cortisol that failed to suppress on overnight dexamethasone administration and an elevated testosterone level. Based on clinical and imaging findings, a presumptive diagnosis of ACC was made. She underwent open adrenalectomy. Pathology revealed ACC with free margins (R0 resection).

SUMMARY

Primary and metastatic cancers involving the adrenal gland are uncommonly encountered in most surgical practices. Patients known or suspected of having such tumors warrant thoughtful consideration of relevant details of their history, physical, biochemical, and imaging evaluation in determining the need for operative intervention and the optimal surgical approach. Selected patients with adrenal lesions potentially representing primary malignancy (<6 cm in size with indeterminate imaging findings) can safely undergo a minimally invasive operation in experienced hands, provided standard oncologic principles are adhered to. It seems reasonable to offer selected patients with isolated metastatic disease to the adrenal gland surgical resection, and MIS via PRA or LA is the preferred approach when anatomically feasible (ie, moderately sized tumor without local-regional invasion). Finally, primary ACC should be removed using an open surgical approach, with a focus on complete en bloc resection. MIS adrenalectomy for ACC should generally continue to be avoided due to the risk of poorer associated outcomes, including tumor capsular disruption with associated incomplete resection, positive resection margins, and risk of early local-regional recurrence and peritoneal carcinomatosis.

REFERENCES

1. Gagner M, Lacroix A, Bolte E. Laparoscopic adrenalectomy in Cushing's syndrome and pheochromocytoma. N Engl J Med 1992;327(14):1033.
2. Bittner JG, Gershuni VM, Matthews BD, et al. Risk factors affecting operative approach, conversion, and morbidity for adrenalectomy: a single-institution series of 402 patients. Surg Endosc 2013;27(7):2342–50.
3. Brunt LM, Doherty GM, Norton JA, et al. Laparoscopic adrenalectomy compared to open adrenalectomy for benign adrenal neoplasms. J Am Coll Surg 1996;183(1):1–10.
4. Gagner M, Pomp A, Heniford BT, et al. Laparoscopic adrenalectomy: lessons learned from 100 consecutive procedures. Ann Surg 1997;226(3):238–46 [discussion: 246–7].
5. Kiernan CM, Shinall MC Jr, Mendez W, et al. Influence of adrenal pathology on perioperative outcomes: a multi-institutional analysis. Am J Surg 2014;208(4):619–25.
6. Lee J, El-Tamer M, Schifftner T, et al. Open and laparoscopic adrenalectomy: analysis of the National Surgical Quality Improvement Program. J Am Coll Surg 2008;206(5):953–9 [discussion: 959–61].
7. Smith CD, Weber CJ, Amerson JR. Laparoscopic adrenalectomy: new gold standard. World J Surg 1999;23(4):389–96.
8. Cooper AB, Habra MA, Grubbs EG, et al. Does laparoscopic adrenalectomy jeopardize oncologic outcomes for patients with adrenocortical carcinoma? Surg Endosc 2013;27(11):4026–32.
9. Miller BS, Ammori JB, Gauger PG, et al. Laparoscopic resection is inappropriate in patients with known or suspected adrenocortical carcinoma. World J Surg 2010;34(6):1380–5.
10. Gonzalez RJ, Shapiro S, Sarlis N, et al. Laparoscopic resection of adrenal cortical carcinoma: a cautionary note. Surgery 2005;138(6):1078–85 [discussion: 1085–76].
11. Leboulleux S, Deandreis D, Al Ghuzlan A, et al. Adrenocortical carcinoma: is the surgical approach a risk factor of peritoneal carcinomatosis? Eur J Endocrinol 2010;162(6):1147–53.
12. Murphy MM, Witkowski ER, Ng SC, et al. Trends in adrenalectomy: a recent national review. Surg Endosc 2010;24(10):2518–26.
13. Sood A, Majumder K, Kachroo N, et al. Adverse event rates, timing of complications, and the impact of specialty on outcomes following adrenal surgery: an analysis of 30-day outcome data from the american college of surgeons national surgical quality improvement program (ACS-NSQIP). Urology 2016;90:62–8.

14. Calcatera NA, Hsiung-Wang C, Suss NR, et al. Minimally invasive adrenalectomy for adrenocortical carcinoma: five-year trends and predictors of conversion. World J Surg 2018;42(2):473–81.
15. Zeiger MA, Thompson GB, Duh QY, et al. American Association of Clinical Endocrinologists and American Association of Endocrine Surgeons Medical Guidelines for the Management of Adrenal Incidentalomas: executive summary of recommendations. Endocr Pract 2009;15(5):450–3.
16. Icard P, Goudet P, Charpenay C, et al. Adrenocortical carcinomas: surgical trends and results of a 253-patient series from the French Association of Endocrine Surgeons study group. World J Surg 2001;25(7):891–7.
17. Margonis GA, Kim Y, Tran TB, et al. Outcomes after resection of cortisol-secreting adrenocortical carcinoma. Am J Surg 2016;211(6):1106–13.
18. NIH state-of-the-science statement on management of the clinically inapparent adrenal mass ("incidentaloma"). NIH Consens State Sci Statements 2002;19(2): 1–25.
19. Lenert JT, Barnett CC Jr, Kudelka AP, et al. Evaluation and surgical resection of adrenal masses in patients with a history of extra-adrenal malignancy. Surgery 2001;130(6):1060–7.
20. Casola G, Nicolet V, vanSonnenberg E, et al. Unsuspected pheochromocytoma: risk of blood-pressure alterations during percutaneous adrenal biopsy. Radiology 1986;159(3):733–5.
21. McCorkell SJ, Niles NL. Fine-needle aspiration of catecholamine-producing adrenal masses: a possibly fatal mistake. AJR Am J Roentgenol 1985;145(1):113–4.
22. Young WF Jr. Clinical practice. The incidentally discovered adrenal mass. N Engl J Med 2007;356(6):601–10.
23. Boland GW, Lee MJ, Gazelle GS, et al. Characterization of adrenal masses using unenhanced CT: an analysis of the CT literature. AJR Am J Roentgenol 1998; 171(1):201–4.
24. Young WF Jr. Conventional imaging in adrenocortical carcinoma: update and perspectives. Horm Cancer 2011;2(6):341–7.
25. Mazzaglia PJ. Radiographic evaluation of nonfunctioning adrenal neoplasms. Surg Clin North Am 2014;94(3):625–42.
26. Blake MA, Kalra MK, Sweeney AT, et al. Distinguishing benign from malignant adrenal masses: multi-detector row CT protocol with 10-minute delay. Radiology 2006;238(2):578–85.
27. Sangwaiya MJ, Boland GW, Cronin CG, et al. Incidental adrenal lesions: accuracy of characterization with contrast-enhanced washout multidetector CT–10-minute delayed imaging protocol revisited in a large patient cohort. Radiology 2010;256(2):504–10.
28. Elsayes KM, Emad-Eldin S, Morani AC, et al. Practical approach to adrenal imaging. Radiol Clin North Am 2017;55(2):279–301.
29. Bednarski BK, Habra MA, Phan A, et al. Borderline resectable adrenal cortical carcinoma: a potential role for preoperative chemotherapy. World J Surg 2014; 38(6):1318–27.
30. Kardar AH. Rupture of adrenal carcinoma after biopsy. J Urol 2001;166(3):984.
31. Quayle FJ, Spitler JA, Pierce RA, et al. Needle biopsy of incidentally discovered adrenal masses is rarely informative and potentially hazardous. Surgery 2007; 142(4):497–502 [discussion: 502–4].
32. Mazzaglia PJ, Monchik JM. Limited value of adrenal biopsy in the evaluation of adrenal neoplasm: a decade of experience. Arch Surg 2009;144(5):465–70.

33. Stefanidis D, Goldfarb M, Kercher KW, et al. SAGES guidelines for minimally invasive treatment of adrenal pathology. Surg Endosc 2013;27(11):3960–80.
34. Anderson KL Jr, Thomas SM, Adam MA, et al. Each procedure matters: threshold for surgeon volume to minimize complications and decrease cost associated with adrenalectomy. Surgery 2018;163(1):157–64.
35. Lindeman B, Hashimoto DA, Bababekov YJ, et al. Fifteen years of adrenalectomies: impact of specialty training and operative volume. Surgery 2018; 163(1):150–6.
36. Barczynski M, Konturek A, Nowak W. Randomized clinical trial of posterior retroperitoneoscopic adrenalectomy versus lateral transperitoneal laparoscopic adrenalectomy with a 5-year follow-up. Ann Surg 2014;260(5):740–7 [discussion: 747–8].
37. Chai YJ, Yu HW, Song RY, et al. Lateral transperitoneal adrenalectomy versus posterior retroperitoneoscopic adrenalectomy for benign adrenal gland disease: randomized controlled trial at a single tertiary medical center. Ann Surg 2017. [Epub ahead of print].
38. Callender GG, Kennamer DL, Grubbs EG, et al. Posterior retroperitoneoscopic adrenalectomy. Adv Surg 2009;43:147–57.
39. Lombardi CP, Raffaelli M, De Crea C, et al. Endoscopic adrenalectomy: is there an optimal operative approach? Results of a single-center case-control study. Surgery 2008;144(6):1008–14 [discussion: 1014–5].
40. Walz MK, Alesina PF, Wenger FA, et al. Posterior retroperitoneoscopic adrenalectomy–results of 560 procedures in 520 patients. Surgery 2006;140(6): 943–8 [discussion: 948–50].
41. Berber E, Tellioglu G, Harvey A, et al. Comparison of laparoscopic transabdominal lateral versus posterior retroperitoneal adrenalectomy. Surgery 2009;146(4): 621–5 [discussion: 625–6].
42. Lam KY, Lo CY. Metastatic tumours of the adrenal glands: a 30-year experience in a teaching hospital. Clin Endocrinol 2002;56(1):95–101.
43. Lee JE, Evans DB, Hickey RC, et al. Unknown primary cancer presenting as an adrenal mass: frequency and implications for diagnostic evaluation of adrenal incidentalomas. Surgery 1998;124(6):1115–22.
44. Moreno P, de la Quintana Basarrate A, Musholt TJ, et al. Adrenalectomy for solid tumor metastases: results of a multicenter European study. Surgery 2013;154(6): 1215–22 [discussion: 1222–3].
45. Romero Arenas MA, Sui D, Grubbs EG, et al. Adrenal metastectomy is safe in selected patients. World J Surg 2014;38(6):1336–42.
46. Strong VE, D'Angelica M, Tang L, et al. Laparoscopic adrenalectomy for isolated adrenal metastasis. Ann Surg Oncol 2007;14(12):3392–400.
47. Glenn JA, Kiernan CM, Yen TW, et al. Management of suspected adrenal metastases at 2 academic medical centers. Am J Surg 2016;211(4):664–70.
48. Kim SH, Brennan MF, Russo P, et al. The role of surgery in the treatment of clinically isolated adrenal metastasis. Cancer 1998;82(2):389–94.
49. Mittendorf EA, Lim SJ, Schacherer CW, et al. Melanoma adrenal metastasis: natural history and surgical management. Am J Surg 2008;195(3):363–8 [discussion: 368–9].
50. Vazquez BJ, Richards ML, Lohse CM, et al. Adrenalectomy improves outcomes of selected patients with metastatic carcinoma. World J Surg 2012;36(6):1400–5.
51. Harisinghani MG, Maher MM, Hahn PF, et al. Predictive value of benign percutaneous adrenal biopsies in oncology patients. Clin Radiol 2002;57(10):898–901.

52. Mansmann G, Lau J, Balk E, et al. The clinically inapparent adrenal mass: update in diagnosis and management. Endocr Rev 2004;25(2):309–40.
53. Dickson PV, Jimenez C, Chisholm GB, et al. Posterior retroperitoneoscopic adrenalectomy: a contemporary American experience. J Am Coll Surg 2011;212(4): 659–65 [discussion: 665–7].
54. Kahramangil B, Berber E. Comparison of posterior retroperitoneal and transabdominal lateral approaches in robotic adrenalectomy: an analysis of 200 cases. Surg Endosc 2018;32(4):1984–9.
55. Perrier ND, Kennamer DL, Bao R, et al. Posterior retroperitoneoscopic adrenalectomy: preferred technique for removal of benign tumors and isolated metastases. Ann Surg 2008;248(4):666–74.
56. Puccini M, Panicucci E, Candalise V, et al. The role of laparoscopic resection of metastases to adrenal glands. Gland Surg 2017;6(4):350–4.
57. Sarela AI, Murphy I, Coit DG, et al. Metastasis to the adrenal gland: the emerging role of laparoscopic surgery. Ann Surg Oncol 2003;10(10):1191–6.
58. Else T, Kim AC, Sabolch A, et al. Adrenocortical carcinoma. Endocr Rev 2014; 35(2):282–326.
59. Varghese J, Habra MA. Update on adrenocortical carcinoma management and future directions. Curr Opin Endocrinol Diabetes Obes 2017;24(3):208–14.
60. Fassnacht M, Allolio B. Clinical management of adrenocortical carcinoma. Best Pract Res Clin Endocrinol Metab 2009;23(2):273–89.
61. Dackiw AP, Lee JE, Gagel RF, et al. Adrenal cortical carcinoma. World J Surg 2001;25(7):914–26.
62. Grubbs EG, Callender GG, Xing Y, et al. Recurrence of adrenal cortical carcinoma following resection: surgery alone can achieve results equal to surgery plus mitotane. Ann Surg Oncol 2010;17(1):263–70.
63. Pommier RF, Brennan MF. An eleven-year experience with adrenocortical carcinoma. Surgery 1992;112(6):963–70 [discussion: 970–1].
64. Brix D, Allolio B, Fenske W, et al. Laparoscopic versus open adrenalectomy for adrenocortical carcinoma: surgical and oncologic outcome in 152 patients. Eur Urol 2010;58(4):609–15.
65. Lee CW, Salem AI, Schneider DF, et al. Minimally invasive resection of adrenocortical carcinoma: a multi-institutional study of 201 patients. J Gastrointest Surg 2017;21(2):352–62.
66. Lombardi CP, Raffaelli M, De Crea C, et al. Open versus endoscopic adrenalectomy in the treatment of localized (stage I/II) adrenocortical carcinoma: results of a multiinstitutional Italian survey. Surgery 2012;152(6):1158–64.
67. Mpaili E, Moris D, Tsilimigras DI, et al. Laparoscopic versus open adrenalectomy for localized/locally advanced primary adrenocortical carcinoma (ENSAT I-III) in adults: is margin-free (R0) resection the key surgical factor that dictates outcome?-A review of the literature. J Laparoendosc Adv Surg Tech A 2018; 28(4):408–14.
68. Porpiglia F, Fiori C, Daffara F, et al. Retrospective evaluation of the outcome of open versus laparoscopic adrenalectomy for stage I and II adrenocortical cancer. Eur Urol 2010;57(5):873–8.
69. Fassnacht M, Arlt W, Bancos I, et al. Management of adrenal incidentalomas: European Society of Endocrinology Clinical Practice Guideline in collaboration with the European Network for the Study of Adrenal Tumors. Eur J Endocrinol 2016; 175(2):G1–34.
70. Bilimoria KY, Shen WT, Elaraj D, et al. Adrenocortical carcinoma in the United States: treatment utilization and prognostic factors. Cancer 2008;113(11):3130–6.

71. Reibetanz J, Jurowich C, Erdogan I, et al. Impact of lymphadenectomy on the oncologic outcome of patients with adrenocortical carcinoma. Ann Surg 2012; 255(2):363–9.
72. Gaujoux S, Brennan MF. Recommendation for standardized surgical management of primary adrenocortical carcinoma. Surgery 2012;152(1):123–32.
73. Huynh KT, Lee DY, Lau BJ, et al. Impact of laparoscopic adrenalectomy on overall survival in patients with nonmetastatic adrenocortical carcinoma. J Am Coll Surg 2016;223(3):485–92.
74. Ayala-Ramirez M, Jasim S, Feng L, et al. Adrenocortical carcinoma: clinical outcomes and prognosis of 330 patients at a tertiary care center. Eur J Endocrinol 2013;169(6):891–9.
75. Fassnacht M, Johanssen S, Fenske W, et al. Improved survival in patients with stage II adrenocortical carcinoma followed up prospectively by specialized centers. J Clin Endocrinol Metab 2010;95(11):4925–32.
76. Hermsen IG, Kerkhofs TM, den Butter G, et al. Surgery in adrenocortical carcinoma: Importance of national cooperation and centralized surgery. Surgery 2012;152(1):50–6.

Minimally Invasive Techniques in Urology

Jairam R. Eswara, MD*, Dicken S. Ko, MD

KEYWORDS

- Urology • Renal cancer • Bladder cancer • Prostate cancer • Robotic surgery

KEY POINTS

- The adoption of robotic techniques has led to an increase in the number of partial nephrectomies done nationwide.
- Partial nephrectomies have more positive outcomes than open partial nephrectomies, comparatively.
- Robotic cystectomy has been shown noninferior to open cystectomy in terms of complications and oncologic outcomes.
- When robotic prostatectomy is compared with open prostatectomy, the results are equivalent or possibly superior with regard to postoperative erectile function and urinary continence.

INTRODUCTION

With the advent of robotic-assisted laparoscopy to offset the difficulties of conventional laparoscopy, the use of minimally invasive techniques for urologic has increased.[1–3] Adoption of robotic surgery in urology, like many new technologies, was early and quick. From natural orifice surgery to fiber optics and new energy transfer methods to conventional laparoscopy and now robotics, urologic surgeons have been early adopters of new techniques. Much of the development of robotic technique has been tied to urologic surgery given the improved visibility for pelvic surgery.

Although the costs have made adoption of robotic systems somewhat less worldwide, the rapid availability of robotic-assisted laparoscopy in the United States and parts of Europe has led to refinement of technique in these regions. Over the past several years, newer data have shown the noninferiority of robotic techniques in urologic oncology, if not outright superiority.

Disclosure: The authors have nothing to disclose.
Department of Surgery, Division of Urology, St. Elizabeth's Hospital, Tufts University School of Medicine, 736 Cambridge Street, Brighton, MA 02135, USA
* Corresponding author.
E-mail address: jeswara@bwh.harvard.edu

RENAL CANCER

With the advantages of robotic surgery clear from prostate surgery, its use began to spread to other urologic malignancies. Although laparoscopic renal surgery had been performed since the early 1990s, robotic renal surgery offered some clear benefits, particularly for partial nephrectomies.[4] Superior visualization as well as articulated robotic wrists add to the technical ease of mass enucleation given the constraint of warm ischemia time. Despite these advantages, however, there has been some debate regarding the actual advantage of nephron-sparing techniques.

Partial Nephrectomy

In 2016, a retrospective review was published comparing 1800 open partial nephrectomies (OPNs) and robotic partial nephrectomies (RPNs).[5] The 2 groups had comparable nephrometry scores, although the robotic group had slightly smaller tumors (33 mm vs 40 mm; $P<.001$). When comparing the 2 groups, the OPN cohort had a higher complication rate (29% vs 18%; $P<.001$), greater blood loss, and more frequent hemorrhagic complications (12% vs 7%; $P<.001$). Also, OPN was associated with a longer warm ischemia time (18.6 min vs 15.7 min; $P<.001$) and longer hospital stay (10.1 days vs 4.7 days; $P<.001$). Oncologic outcomes were the same. The investigators concluded that where was a clear advantage to RPNs compared with OPNs.

A meta-analysis from 2016 demonstrated a benefit for RPNs compared with laparoscopic partial nephrectomies.[6] A total of 4919 patients from 25 studies were included, and, despite patients in the robotic group having larger tumors and higher nephrometry scores, they had lower rates of conversion to open, any complications, major (Clavien $\geq$3) complications, and positive margins and shorter warm ischemia time. Operative times and blood loss were similar as were postoperative estimated glomerular filtration rates. The investigators concluded that RPN is superior to laparoscopic partial nephrectomy with regard to perioperative outcomes and morbidity.

As RPNs have proliferated, so has the treatment, or overtreatment, of small renal masses. A study examining the National Cancer Database (NCDB) sought to determine the effect.[7] From 2010 to 2014, they found that the rate of increase in RPN and radical nephrectomy outpaced that of active surveillance for small renal masses (<4 cm). This trend also was seen among those older than 75 years and those with Charlson index 2 or greater. This raised the concern that the adoption of robotic techniques is leading to overtreatment of small renal masses among the elderly and infirm.

A meta-analysis from 2018 looked at the impact of host factors on the outcomes of RPN.[8] The analysis included 41 studies totaling 10,506 patients. Tumor factors associated with worse outcomes included tumors larger than 4 cm and hilar tumor, as were patient factors, such as obesity. Another study from Cleveland Clinic in 2017 found that RPN was associated with higher rates of negative surgical margins, absence of perioperative outcomes, greater than or equal to 80% renal function preservation, and no chronic kidney disease upstaging.[9]

Radical Nephrectomy Versus Partial Nephrectomy

Two recent studies have differing views regarding the benefits of partial nephrectomy compared with radical nephrectomy, albeit in select cohorts. An NCDB study published in *Cancer* in 2018 suggested that partial nephrectomy for masses larger than 4 cm was not associated with a survival advantage compared with radical nephrectomy in the elderly.[10] The study did find, however, an advantage among all patients who underwent partial nephrectomy for T1 or T2 disease.

Another study using the Surveillance, Epidemiology, and End Results database and National Inpatient Sample used propensity score matching to determine the effect of partial nephrectomy compared radical nephrectomy for patients with metastatic disease.[11] Among patients from 2004 to 2013, 217 of 5171 patients with metastatic renal cell carcinoma underwent partial nephrectomy. Multivariate logistic regression showed that partial nephrectomy was associated with lower rates of blood transfusions, intraoperative surgical complications, and other-cause mortality. No difference was seen in overall complications or in-hospital mortality.

BLADDER CANCER

Over the past decade, robot-assisted radical cystectomy (RARC) has grown in use as an alternative to open radical cystectomy (ORC). Patients with bladder cancer often have multiple comorbidities, and the surgeries themselves are complex and fraught with complications. More recently, several studies have assessed the outcomes of ORC and RARC.

A large retrospective series using the NCDB compared the effectiveness of ORC and RARC.[12] The study compared patients who underwent the surgeries between 2010 and 2013 and found that RARC was noninferior in several parameters. With regard to positive surgical margins (10.7% vs 9.3%; $P = .10$) and 30-day and 90-day postoperative complications (2.8% vs 1.4% and 6.7% vs 4.8%, respectively), the rates between the 2 groups were not statistically different. With regard to the rates of pelvic lymph node dissection, median lymph node count, length of stay, and overall survival, RARC was found superior, however. Although only 1 in 4 cystectomies was done robotically during this time period, the advantages of the robotic approach were clear.

Perhaps the most important study to compare these 2 modalities is the RAZOR study whose results were published in *Lancet* in 2018.[13] Between 2011 and 2014, 350 patients were randomized to either ORC or RARC as a noninferiority trial. Adverse events were noted in 69% of the ORC group and 67% of the RARC group. Importantly, 2-year progression-free survival was 71.6% and 72.3% in the ORC and RARC groups, respectively. The most common complications were urinary tract infection (26% in the ORC group and 35% in the RARC group) and postoperative ileus (20% in the ORC group and 22% in the RARC group). This study shows the noninferiority of robotic-assisted radical cystectomy.

A recent retrospective study conducted by the International Robotic Cystectomy Consortium compared open and robotic intracorporeal urinary diversions.[14] The study found that patients who underwent an intracorporeal urinary diversion had a shorter operative time (357 min vs 400 min; $P<.001$), less blood loss (300 mL vs 350 mL; $P<.001$), and fewer blood transfusions (4% vs 19%; $P<.001$). They did experience more high-grade complications (13% vs 10%; $P = .02$). As the number of intracorporeal conduits has increased with time, the rate of high-grade complications has decreased with time.

PROSTATE CANCER

The benefits of minimally invasive prostatectomy over open prostatectomy (OP) have been well documented in the literature. Several studies have reported less blood loss during robot-associated laparoscopic prostatectomy (RALP).[15,16] Control over the dorsal venous complex is the critical step to ensuring minimal blood loss during prostatectomy, and laparoscopic visualization is advantageous. In addition, the tamponade of pneumoperitoneum is likely helpful in minimizing blood loss.

Postoperative pain seems comparable between robotic and open cohorts, likely due to the relatively less painful infraumbilical incision for the open procedure.[17,18] Older data suggested an equivalent postoperative length of stay; however, more recent data suggest a shorter length of stay with RALP.[19–21]

The risk of urinary incontinence and erectile dysfunction after prostatectomy remains a concern, regardless of technique. A cohort study from the National Health Service in England compared patients who underwent OP (n = 6873), laparoscopic prostatectomy (LP) (n =5479), and robotic prostatectomy (n = 4947) from 2008 to 2012.[22] In this study, men who underwent RALP had the lowest rates of urinary complications (OP 19.1% vs LP 15.8% vs RALP 10.5%). In their series, men who underwent robotic prostatectomy also had the lowest rate of bladder neck contractures and urethral strictures (OP 6.9% vs LP 5.7% vs RALP 3.3%). They concluded that men who underwent RALP had superior urinary outcomes.

Another study of patient reported outcomes from the Mayo Clinic and Massachusetts General Hospital compared the 3 modalities.[23] The study was from 2009 to 2012 with a median follow-up of 30.5 months. The study included 441 patients who underwent OP, 156 who underwent LP, and 1089 who underwent RALP. This analysis found no statistical difference among the 3 groups with regard to urinary dysfunction (OP 5.8%, LRP 5.1%, and RALP 6.8%; $P = .62$), or erectile dysfunction (OP 37.2%, LRP 36.1%, and RALP 37.5%; $P = .95$).

A 2016 study from Milan examined the rates of orgasmic dysfunction after OP and RALP.[24] This series found a significantly lower rate of climacturia and painful orgasm among the patients who underwent RALP in their cohort. A follow-up study by the same group in 2018 found that patients who underwent RALP reported a lower risk of postoperative penile morphometric alterations (penile curvature or shortening) compared with those who underwent OP (odds ratio [OR] 0.38).[25]

One of the few randomized controlled trials comparing OP and RALP was published in 2018.[26] It compared urinary function, erectile function, and oncologic outcomes. At the 24-month time point, there was no significant difference between the 2 groups with regard to urinary or sexual function. Superiority testing of the biochemical recurrence rates suggested a better outcome in the robotic group, but equivalence testing of progression on imaging showed no statistical difference. The investigators conclude the main benefit of RALP is related to its "minimally invasive nature."[26]

A large database study using a nationwide sample compared 90-day complication rates between OP and RALP using the Premier hospital database.[3] They found that patients who underwent RALP were less likely to experience any complications (OR 0.68; $P<.001$), have a prolonged hospitalization (OR 0.28; $P<.001$), or receive blood products (OR 0.33; $P = .002$). They found that the 90-day direct hospital costs were higher, however in the RALP group, $4528 more on average. Another large database analysis compared the rates of small bowel obstruction after OP and RALP using the SEER-Medicare database.[27] With a median follow-up of 76 months for the OP cohort and 45 months for the RALP cohort, there was no statistical difference in rates between the 2 groups.

SUMMARY

Robotic surgery for urologic oncology has proliferated over the past several decades, and robotic techniques have become integral to all aspects of the field. Recent data have shown improved outcomes with robotic techniques as a result of greater surgeon experience. Renal surgery, in particular the partial nephrectomy, has benefited from the adoption of robotic technology. Not only has it made the procedure safer but also more common in the United States.[6] Although radical cystectomies still remain a morbid procedure, the growing adoption of robotic-assisted radical cystectomies has led to comparable outcomes in a randomized controlled trial and superior outcomes in well-done retrospective studies.[12,13] Because most prostatectomies in the United States are now done robotically, the data here are perhaps the strongest. A randomized controlled trial showed there was no difference between OP and robotic prostatectomy with regard to erectile and urinary function, but retrospective studies have suggested most perioperative outcomes are improved with the robotic technique.[3,26,28] As implementation of robotic techniques continues to increase, it is likely that the outcomes for all of these procedures will continue to improve.

REFERENCES

1. Cheung H, Wang Y, Chang SL, et al. Adoption of robot-assisted partial nephrectomies: a population-based analysis of U.S. surgeons from 2004 to 2013. J Endourol 2017;31:886.
2. Chang SL, Kibel AS, Brooks JD, et al. The impact of robotic surgery on the surgical management of prostate cancer in the USA. BJU Int 2015;115:929.
3. Leow JJ, Chang SL, Meyer CP, et al. Robot-assisted versus open radical prostatectomy: a contemporary analysis of an all-payer discharge database. Eur Urol 2016;70:837.
4. Clayman RV, Kavoussi LR, Soper NJ, et al. Laparoscopic nephrectomy. N Engl J Med 1991;324:1370.
5. Peyronnet B, Seisen T, Oger E, et al. Comparison of 1800 robotic and open partial nephrectomies for renal tumors. Ann Surg Oncol 2016;23:4277.
6. Leow JJ, Heah NH, Chang SL, et al. Outcomes of robotic versus laparoscopic partial nephrectomy: an updated meta-analysis of 4,919 patients. J Urol 2016; 196:1371.
7. Shah PH, Alom MA, Leibovich BC, et al. The temporal association of robotic surgical diffusion with overtreatment of the small renal mass. J Urol 2018;200:981.
8. Cacciamani GE, Gill T, Medina L, et al. Impact of host factors on robotic partial nephrectomy outcomes: comprehensive systematic review and meta-analysis. J Urol 2018;200:716.
9. Maurice MJ, Ramirez D, Kara Ö, et al. Optimum outcome achievement in partial nephrectomy for T1 renal masses: a contemporary analysis of open and robot-assisted cases. BJU Int 2017;120:537.
10. Ristau BT, Handorf EA, Cahn DB, et al. Partial nephrectomy is not associated with an overall survival advantage over radical nephrectomy in elderly patients with stage Ib-II renal masses: an analysis of the national cancer data base. Cancer 2018;124:3839.
11. Mazzone E, Nazzani S, Preisser F, et al. Partial nephrectomy seems to confer a survival benefit relative to radical nephrectomy in metastatic renal cell carcinoma. Cancer Epidemiol 2018;56:118.
12. Hanna N, Leow JJ, Sun M, et al. Comparative effectiveness of robot-assisted vs. open radical cystectomy. Urol Oncol 2018;36:88.e1-9.
13. Parekh DJ, Reis IM, Castle EP, et al. Robot-assisted radical cystectomy versus open radical cystectomy in patients with bladder cancer (RAZOR): an open-label, randomised, phase 3, non-inferiority trial. Lancet 2018;391:2525.
14. Hussein AA, May PR, Jing Z, et al. Outcomes of intracorporeal urinary diversion after robot-assisted radical cystectomy: results from the international robotic cystectomy consortium. J Urol 2018;199:1302.

15. Ficarra V, Novara G, Artibani W, et al. Retropubic, laparoscopic, and robot-assisted radical prostatectomy: a systematic review and cumulative analysis of comparative studies. Eur Urol 2009;55:1037.

16. Kordan Y, Barocas DA, Altamar HO, et al. Comparison of transfusion requirements between open and robotic-assisted laparoscopic radical prostatectomy. BJU Int 2010;106:1036.

17. Webster TM, Herrell SD, Chang SS, et al. Robotic assisted laparoscopic radical prostatectomy versus retropubic radical prostatectomy: a prospective assessment of postoperative pain. J Urol 2005;174:912.

18. Tewari A, Srivasatava A, Menon M, et al. A prospective comparison of radical retropubic and robot-assisted prostatectomy: experience in one institution. BJU Int 2003;92:205.

19. Jackson MA, Bellas N, Siegrist T, et al. Experienced open vs early robotic-assisted laparoscopic radical prostatectomy: a 10-year prospective and retrospective comparison. Urology 2016;91:111.

20. Nelson B, Kaufman M, Broughton G, et al. Comparison of length of hospital stay between radical retropubic prostatectomy and robotic assisted laparoscopic prostatectomy. J Urol 2007;177:929.

21. Rocco B, Matei DV, Melegari S, et al. Robotic vs open prostatectomy in a laparoscopically naive centre: a matched-pair analysis. BJU Int 2009;104:991.

22. Sujenthiran A, Nossiter J, Parry M, et al. National cohort study comparing severe medium-term urinary complications after robot-assisted vs laparoscopic vs retropubic open radical prostatectomy. BJU Int 2018;121:445.

23. Gershman B, Psutka SP, McGovern FJ, et al. Patient-reported functional outcomes following open, laparoscopic, and robotic assisted radical prostatectomy performed by high-volume surgeons at high-volume hospitals. Eur Urol Focus 2016;2:172.

24. Capogrosso P, Ventimiglia E, Serino A, et al. Orgasmic dysfunction after robot-assisted versus open radical prostatectomy. Eur Urol 2016;70:223.

25. Capogrosso P, Ventimiglia E, Cazzaniga W, et al. Long-term penile morphometric alterations in patients treated with robot-assisted versus open radical prostatectomy. Andrology 2018;6:136.

26. Coughlin GD, Yaxley JW, Chambers SK, et al. Robot-assisted laparoscopic prostatectomy versus open radical retropubic prostatectomy: 24-month outcomes from a randomised controlled study. Lancet Oncol 2018;19:1051.

27. Loeb S, Meyer CP, Krasnova A, et al. Risk of small bowel obstruction after robot-assisted vs open radical prostatectomy. J Endourol 2016;30:1291.

28. Leow JJ, Reese SW, Jiang W, et al. Propensity-matched comparison of morbidity and costs of open and robot-assisted radical cystectomies: a contemporary population-based analysis in the United States. Eur Urol 2014;66:569.

Afterword

Brice Gayet, MD, PhD*, David Fuks, MD, PhD

KEYWORDS

- Cancer • Esophagectomy • Hepatectomy • Laparoscopy
- Simulation-based training • Tumor

KEY POINTS

- The physical removal of solid tumors via surgery continues to be the primary method of curative intent treatment.
- Randomized trials have shown that a minimally invasive approach is associated with improved postoperative recovery without compromising oncologic outcomes.
- Diffusion of laparoscopy to complex procedures or even pediatric tumors, has been limited due to technological difficulties, concerns regarding patient and oncologic safety and a long learning curve.
- Additional challenges are rapid technology evolution, resource constrains leading to decreased trainee operative time, and maintenance of expertise in maximally invasive procedures needed for complex clinical scenarios.
- The time when an intervention will be a succession of autonomously performed minimally invasive procedures, helped or even performed by robots, may not be as farfetched as previously believed.

Despite significant improvements over the last several decades in multimodality treatment for cancer, the physical removal of solid tumors via surgery continues to be the primary method of curative intent treatment. Currently, neoadjuvant treatments using modern chemotherapy and novel radiation protocols are used to reduce tumor size or diminish the risk of systemic relapse before removal of the bulk tumor. Aiming for cure, these improvements in the management of solid cancers remain dependent on the ability to remove tumors.

Historically, open surgery through large incisions was the standard approach for surgical procedures to remove cancers. However, the pioneers of colorectal and genitourinary oncologic surgery were able to develop less invasive surgeries with the aid of cameras and via minimal access approaches that led to the field expanding to other areas of surgical oncologic. From initial experimental investigations using animal

Disclosure Statement: The authors have no conflicts of interest and have nothing to disclose.
Department of Digestive, Oncologic and Metabolic Surgery, Institut Mutualiste Montsouris, Université Paris Descartes, 42 Boulevard Jourdan, Paris 75014, France
* Corresponding author.
E-mail address: brice.gayet@imm.fr

models and then applying these findings to patient investigations, the benefits of a laparoscopic approach in the management of cancer became clear. These benefits include improved pain control, rapid postoperative recovery, and improved patient satisfaction. In this setting, a significant number of well-conducted randomized trials have shown that a minimally invasive approach is associated with improved postoperative recovery without compromising oncologic outcomes.

When the field expanded to gastrointestinal malignancies, laparoscopy was initially used for staging to assess for radiographically occult metastatic disease and for resectability in selected patients. Although seemingly a minor procedure, staging laparoscopy helps to avoid nontherapeutic laparotomy in patients with unresectable cancer. It is associated with shorter length of hospital stay and time to adjuvant therapy compared with nontherapeutic laparotomy. However, after the use of laparoscopy for staging and minor procedures, the field of laparoscopic gastrointestinal cancer surgery progressed to complex surgeries such esophagectomies. In this context, a well-designed trial investigating surgical morbidity after esophagectomy for cancer suggests that a laparoscopic approach in itself could improve long-term outcomes. These promising new findings prompted us to develop a randomized controlled trial to better understand the relationship between reduced trauma and cancer recurrence.

With the advancement in laparoscopic gastrointestinal surgery, minimal access surgery expanded to treating children with minimally invasive surgery as adjunctive and definitive surgical treatment for different pediatric tumors. Challenges to minimally invasive surgery for pediatric tumors include a small working space for comparatively large tumors, the need for a large incision for extraction, and the fact that heterogeneity of tumor types defies a uniform approach and that there is often a low case volume per tumor type for most surgeons.

Despite successful application of laparoscopy for complex gastrointestinal malignancies and even pediatric tumors, the diffusion of laparoscopy to more complex procedures such as liver surgery has been limited due to technological difficulties such as the absence of specific laparoscopic devices, concerns regarding patient safety (gas embolism, uncontrollable hemorrhage) and oncologic safety (incomplete resection), and a long learning curve (expertise in both liver and laparoscopic surgery). Hence, it is only in the early-mid 2000s that larger series reporting the safety and feasibility of laparoscopic liver resection were reported. To date, more than 9000 laparoscopic liver resections have been performed and both feasibility and safety of a minimally invasive approach are now largely accepted. The authors' team, having performed one thousand laparoscopic liver resections to date, strongly believes that a clear training pathway is needed. This training pathway should be based on the objectively assessed difficulty of a particular liver resection and result in safe dissemination. Because of concerns for subjectivity when grading the complexity of laparoscopic liver resection, the authors have proposed a new and objective classification of laparoscopic liver resection based on its difficulty. Although it is clear that the modern surgical oncologist requires extensive training in minimally invasive techniques, the increasing constraints on time and resources have led to a new emphasis on finding innovative ways to teach minimally invasive surgical skills, both inside and outside the operating room. Additional challenges are rapid technology evolution, resource constrains leading to decreased trainee operative time, and maintenance of expertise in maximally invasive procedures needed for complex clinical scenarios. In this context, simulation-based training allows trainees to learn technical and nontechnical skills without risking patient safety. It is increasingly being incorporated into surgical training or mandated by certifying bodies. Simulation-based training may lead to excellent skills transfer, with resulting increase in patient safety, procedural efficiency, and cost savings.

In parallel to the innovations in minimal access surgery, the role of endoscopy has drastically evolved over time, both in terms of its diagnostic as well as interventional abilities. Endoscopic placement of luminal stents can be used for palliation or to treat postsurgical complications such as strictures. The role of endoscopy will grow in the future with potentially injectable drug delivery into tumors, as well as advanced drug-eluting stent placements.

This comprehensive update by Surgical Oncology Clinics of North America on Minimally Invasive Cancer Management allows the reader to have an exhaustive overview of the role of minimally invasive approaches to removing solid tumors, palliation, technical innovations (robotic, transluminal surgery or augmented reality), and learning.

When reading these 2 very important parts of Surgical Oncology Clinics of North America, it becomes clear how actively teams are working on future innovations in minimally invasive cancer management. Articles on the increasing role of (1) computer and digital sciences for augmented reality, (2) the use of robotics from the aerodigestive tract to the pelvic floor, and finally (3) surgery by natural orifices highlight this. Although robotics is currently limited to simple endoscopic procedures or telemanipulation with questionable cost-effectiveness, it may become a new standard of care due to robotic platform development with flexible instruments and artificial intelligence. The time when an intervention will be a succession of autonomously performed minimally invasive procedures may not be as farfetched as previously believed and is already the subject of research investigations today.

In conclusion, we have continued to see the introduction of many innovative techniques for the diagnosis and treatment of cancer during the first decade of the twenty-first century. These technical advances have been based on the application of laparoscopic and other minimal access approaches to cancer surgery. This has led to newer methods of cancer resection. The era when robots will be more than simple remote manipulators or when advanced natural orifice endoscopy may be used to remove complex cancers in an oncologically sound way is rapidly approaching. It is important to continue applying high-quality science to these future applications in the form of randomized controlled trials. The data derived from these studies should lead to guidelines that avoid the pitfalls associated with the application of inappropriate oncologic principals. It should always be kept in mind that progress in health care is not about "novelty" or "innovation" itself but about improvement in care or lower costs.

The appropriate application of the technical advances described in these special issues of Surgical Oncology Clinics of North America depends on the individual physicians caring compassionately for their patients who must not forget that technology tends to move faster than science, which moves faster than wisdom.

Moving?

Make sure your subscription moves with you!

To notify us of your new address, find your **Clinics Account Number** (located on your mailing label above your name), and contact customer service at:

Email: journalscustomerservice-usa@elsevier.com

800-654-2452 (subscribers in the U.S. & Canada)
314-447-8871 (subscribers outside of the U.S. & Canada)

Fax number: 314-447-8029

Elsevier Health Sciences Division
Subscription Customer Service
3251 Riverport Lane
Maryland Heights, MO 63043

*To ensure uninterrupted delivery of your subscription, please notify us at least 4 weeks in advance of move.